LOOKING FOR THE CASHCOW

Action Steps to Improve Cash Flow in Medical Group Practices

Thomas G. Hajny

Edited by Kerstin B. Lynam

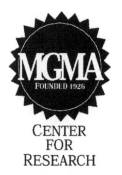

CENTER
FOR
RESEARCH

ISBN: 1-56829-022-5

Library of Congress Catalog Card Number: 00-135241

Printed in the United States of America
10 9 8 7 6 5 4 3 2 1

Disclaimer

The MGMA Center for Research, the research and development arm of the Medical Group Management Association (MGMA), prints publications that are intended to provide current and accurate information and are designed to assist readers in becoming more familiar with the subject matter covered. Such publications are distributed with the understanding that the MGMA Center for Research and MGMA do not render any legal, accounting or other professional advice. No representations nor warranties are made concerning the application of legal or other principles discussed by the author to any specific fact situation, nor is any prediction made concerning how any particular judge, government official, or other person will interpret or apply such principles. Specific factual situations should be discussed with professional advisors.

To my dearest companion, my best friend, and my love
— my wife Charlene

Thomas G. Hajny
Bayside, Wisconsin, June 2000

Acknowledgments

There are many people to thank, mostly the bright and dedicated physicians and practice managers who have given me most (all?) of the good ideas and strategies in this book. I most profusely thank them for allowing me into their practices and lives. All of you have shown a generosity most unique.

Looking for the Cashcow would have never been born without the inspiration of my friend and mentor, Mr. David Zimmerman of Zimmerman & Associates whose own book *Twelve Key Strategies* provided much of the insight into the chapters on motivation and goal setting. I also thank David for bringing me into the world of the consultant. He has a vision of the consultant as a significant contributor to health care by advising medical groups in effective cash management. This makes consulting not a job but a mission.

While David provided the inspiration, it was my editor — Kerstin Lynam — who brought this book into the light of day. With a good sense of humor and an iron fist, she made sure I kept on schedule. To Kerstin I thank many times over.

And finally I must thank Sara Larch, FACMPE, Chief Operating Officer of University Physicians, Inc. in Baltimore, MD who reviewed *Looking for the Cashcow* and made significant (and numerous) suggestions. Her thorough and exacting recommendations took this workbook to the next level.

In the end the author is humbled by the knowledge of how little I did without the kind and candid support of my friends. Thank you kind friends.

About the Author

Tom Hajny

Tom Hajny provides consulting services to clinics and hospitals for revenue cycle and cash management performance improvement. His health care experience spans over 16 years as a vice-president of consulting for a national health care receivables firm, director of an independent physicians association, financial analyst, managing editor of health care orientated newsletters, and a central business office manager for a large clinic/hospital system. His consulting experience includes projects with large and small health care facilities — from rural clinics to major urban facilities.

Tom is a contributor to the health care discussions with frequent articles in *The Journal of Medical Practice Management*, Healthcare Financial Management Association (HFMA) periodicals, and program presentations on cash management in health care. Tom holds two undergraduate Bachelor of Science degrees — the first from the University of Wisconsin with a major in English and a minor in Philosophy, the second from Edgewood College with a major in Business Administration with emphasis in Accounting.

About the Medical Group Management Association (MGMA) and the MGMA Center for Research

Since its founding in 1926, MGMA has become the leading membership, education and research organization for professionals in medical practice management. MGMA is headquartered in Englewood, Colorado. MGMA's diverse membership includes administrators, CEOs and board members of health systems, physicians in management, office managers and many other management professionals from medical practices of all sizes and types, as well as from integrated health systems, hospital and medical school-affiliated practices and practice management organizations.

Founded in 1973 with funding from the W.K. Kellogg Foundation, the MGMA Center for Research (formerly The MGMA Center for Research in Ambulatory Health Care Administration, CRAHCA), is organized as a 501(c)(3) tax-exempt charitable organization as defined by the Internal Revenue Code. The MGMA Center for Research relies on foundation, corporate and government grants and revenue from education programs, publications and software, as well as interest from its endowment fund and services provided to the MGMA. The MGMA Center for Research endowment fund was established in 1978 and continues to grow through tax-deductible contributions from individuals and corporations.

The MGMA Center for Research conducts health services research, develops measurement tools and conducts educational seminars for the benefit of the entire health care industry. Its mission is to advance the art and science of medical group practice management to improve the health of our communities through health services research based largely in group practices and other health care delivery settings.

About Zimmerman & Associates, LLC

Zimmerman & Associates is a revenue cycle consulting group that has brought financial success to health care providers nationwide. The firm specializes in accelerating cash flow, impacting patient relations and improving revenue cycle operations.

Nearly 300 health care providers have sought out Zimmerman & Associates consulting expertise over the past five years. The last five major consulting assignments resulted in more than $85 million in improvement for the client hospitals.

Chairman David Zimmerman, and his wife Peggy, executive vice president, founded Zimmerman & Associates in 1986. David's professional background includes 17 years in hospital financial management and several years of experience in consumer finance, the Health Care Financial Management Association, Blue Cross and a management consulting firm in Chicago.

For the past 14 years, members of the consulting staff have presented nearly 400 seminars around the nation for health care employees. Several customized training programs have also been developed for specific providers, as well as in-house training packages with videos, leader's guides and workbooks for Business Office and Registration personnel. The firm has also produced audio programs, reports and booklets on topics related to managing accounts receivable.

Zimmerman is the founding publisher of numerous successful newsletters and books, including the *Receivables Report*, the nationally renowned Hospital Accounts Receivable Analysis (*HARA*), and eight other healthcare financial newsletters. He is also the author of ten diverse health care books, including, *Cash is King* and *Unleash the Potential, Unlocking the Mystery of Motivation*.

Returning to the industry, Zimmerman Communications is the health care media group that focuses on improving customer service, collection effectiveness and management of the revenue cycle. Its newsletters include *Customer Service Revolution*, *Collection Expert* and Hospital Receivables Management.

From newsletters to multi-media training programs, benchmarks to annual reports, Z Comm delivers industry products that impact the way health care facilities operate, ultimately improving the bottom line.

As experts in the field, Zimmerman & Associates delivers relevant, timely and real-world advice that is applied in day-to-day health care environments.

By Way of an Introduction...
How to Use *Looking for the Cashcow*

One of the initial struggles an author (and editor) must contend with is how to present the material — how to organize the flow of information in a way that the reader finds usable and useful. Useful! — that's the key word. What information and in what format does the physician or the practice management manager need, desire, and demand in order to take action?

Looking for the Cashcow is unique in that it asks you to step outside your role as a practice manager and become... an outside consultant. An outside consultant who will look at your practice with fresh eyes and compare what is currently being done against a "best practices" model.

Looking for the Cashcow was born out of the notion that certain revenue cycle activities — properly implemented — will bring to a practice more cash through revenue recapture, faster turnaround from service to collection, lower bad debt expense, higher productivity from your staff, while enhancing patient service. The model presented in this book does not involve an infinite number of functions nor are they necessarily difficult to grasp in concept. Where most practices fall down is in the implementation — the action!

When you open this book please do so with the mindset of taking action. Instead of presenting the materials in traditional "chapters," I tried to underline the intended "action" approach by calling the 12 sections "key action steps." Each key action step introduces an area of the revenue cycle to give you the required information to change your practice. At the end of each key action step is a series of questions to ask yourself and a "to do" list. Some of the to-do's you can do immediately, others you will need to plan out, communicate thoroughly and read the final chapters on creating an action plan, setting goals, and providing the motivational environment in which to achieve ultimate success.

If, after you have completed reading *Looking for the Cashcow*, you have not implemented any changes to your practice, then one of three things has taken place. The first consideration is you already run a great shop and *Looking for the Cashcow* has confirmed this fact. Second, I have let you down and not presented the material in a clear and useful manner. The third option is that you have backed down from the stimulating and exciting challenge of doing what you know is right – either because of "politics" or the "culture" or ...? It is my hope *Looking for the Cashcow* gives you the information and the determination to sally forth into battle, courageous in your righteousness. And remember... if not you, Who? If not now, When?

Sincerely,
Tom

Table of Contents

Key Action Step 1
DEVELOP A STRATEGY!

Receivables management need not be a mystifying and frustrating science. What is needed are comprehensive strategies which address short-term cash needs and long-term performance improvements. In this first strategy, the need to develop and analyze the key receivable indicators is explored.

The call which produces an instant headache

You just received a call from the practice's accountant and things aren't good. It appears "Our Practice's" cash is down and account receivables are up. "These trends have been ongoing for the last six months," she says, "Something needs to be done." You put down the phone and take a deep breath. You think, "I need to do something, but what?" You review all the things *being done*: staff is working accounts — *when they have time*. The managed care firm who has had trouble making payments on a timely basis is *still* holding your cash. That other insurance company just went through a computer conversion and they think they will catch up (with payments) — *soon*. One of the staff is out for two weeks with a bad back, so patient follow-up is a *"little behind"* and on and on and on…

You've been here before and you realize putting out the fire of the day — or week or month — is not the answer. What you are looking for is a process to address this on-going, seemingly never-ending problem. It is time to try a different approach.

What to do? Know the numbers of receivables management

Just as in the pursuit of a medical diagnosis, bringing accounts receivable (and cash) back to health begins with the facts. These statistical "facts" will not only form the basis of your recommendations for performance improvements, but the statistics will also be the basis for your goal setting and monitoring program. These *key indicators* have to become part of your normal, continuous review process.

Net charges to cash collections

The most important statistic you need to review is **Cash Collections.** Cash collection is the movement of receivables into a commodity you can use — cash. Cash is, after all, the point of having a receivables system. To know how efficient your system is, you will need to trend cash collections and *net charges* over the last twelve months

NOTE: *Net charges (or net revenue) are the usual and customary charges of the practice less any "contractual allowances." Contractual allowances are those discounts which are granted based on managed care agreements or governmental regulation.*

In the best of all-possible worlds (and assuming a constant net charge), your cash and net charges trend lines should stay close and parallel.

In Exhibit 1.1, "Our Practice" is having trouble meeting its expected cash collections. The "cash gap" has been widening since June and there is no indication the trend is slowing down. This chart sounds a loud alarm for an immediate cash acceleration program. Because of the severe gap, the entire revenue cycle must be reviewed. Immediate concerns are whether the payers are receiving bills and statements. Concurrently, a "rejected claim" analysis needs to be done to ascertain whether "unclean" claims are delaying "Our Practice's" cash.

Exhibit 1.1 "Our Practice's" net charges versus cash collections

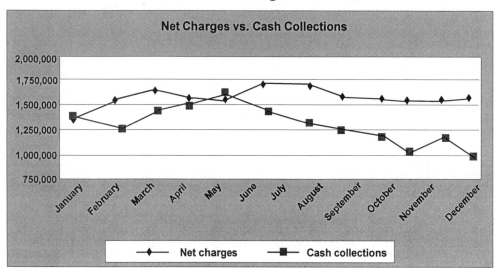

Net Days Revenue Outstanding (NDRO)

This is your second most important indicator:

Net Receivables ÷ (Net Charges ÷ Days in Period)

This statistic indicates the number of days, on average, from the date of service to the collection of cash. Depending on your practice management system, you may have trouble calculating "net." At the time of billing, if you do not write-off contractual allowances (the difference between what you charge and what you *can* be paid), your receivables may be stated as "gross" (charges). In this case, a Gross Day's Revenue Outstanding (GDRO) calculation will work.

Gross Receivables ÷ (Gross Revenue ÷ Days in Period)

This statistic, when compared to peer groups or benchmarks, will provide an insight into how bad is "bad."

In Exhibit 1.2, "Our Practice's" day's revenue outstanding (DRO) of 93.2, just in terms of cash flow, is unacceptable. Unless your vendors let you pay your bills, on average, in 93.2 days, your cash flow is in trouble. In the comparisons, "Our Practice" is far removed from the benchmark performing practices (49.3) and the averages demonstrated by comparable physician size peer groups. The benchmark number indicates the ultimate goal of "Our Practice," while the peer group statistic tells us what should be achievable in the short term. This comparison study reveals there is much work to be done but it doesn't give much insight into where the problems might be found.

Exhibit 1.2 "Our Practice's" days revenue outstanding (DRO)

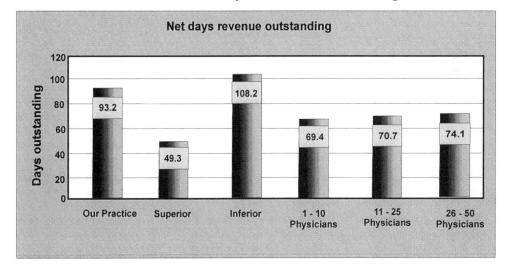

The DRO should also be trended over the last twelve months (24 months would be even better as it allows for an inspection of seasonal fluctuations). This will give you a visual representation of where you are heading and will pinpoint "jumps" which will identify when and possibly what environmental changes occurred.

The example on the following page shows how to calculate "Our Practice's" day's revenue outstanding (DRO) — remember not to mix gross and net revenue and receivables:

$$DRO = \frac{\text{Dollars in accounts receivable}}{\text{One day's charges (revenue)}}$$

$$\text{Day's revenue} = \frac{\text{Total revenue last three months (90 days used for example)}}{\text{Number of days last three months}}$$
$$\text{(90 days used as an example)}$$

Revenue month 1 =   \$1,710,535
Revenue month 2 =   \$1,490,993
Revenue month 3 =   \$1,508,472
Total revenue   \$4,710,000

$$\text{Days revenue} = \frac{\$4,710,000}{90} = \$52,333$$

The calculation for the day's revenue is based on a three months' "rolling average" versus just one month because it "smooths out" any aberrations in revenue. Thus, it is more likely to accurately reflect "Our Practice's" average daily revenues.

Assuming total accounts receivables of \$4,877,436, the DRO is calculated as follows:

$$DRO = \frac{\$4,877,436}{\$52,333} = 93.20$$

What should the DRO be?

Is 93.2 DRO good or bad? Let's ask the question, "What should the DRO be?" Exhibit 1.3 breaks the analysis down by payer, projecting how long a "clean" claim will take to be paid — estimating the time-to-payment based on contract terms or, in the case of government payers, by regulation. The "should be DRO" is calculated by simple multiplication of the payer mix percentage and the DRO ideal. "Our Practice" ideal DRO is the sum of all the DRO mixes.

Exhibit 1.3 Calculation of "Our Practice's" ideal DRO

	Payer Mix	DRO Ideal	DRO Mix
Blue Cross	14%	45	6.3
Commercial	12%	45	5.4
Contract Commercial	12%	45	5.4
Medicaid	6%	35	2.1
Medicare	40%	30	12.0
Workers' compensation	5%	90	4.5
Other	1%	60	0.6
Self-pay	10%	60	6.0
"Our Practice" ideal DRO	100%		**42.3**

Comparing the ideal DRO for "Our Practice" with the actual DRO gives insight on how well (or poorly) "Our Practice" is handling its accounts receivables. How good does 93.2 DRO look now?

Aging reports

An Aged Trial Balance (ATB) is a report generated by your practice management system. The ATB allows the practice to know, by payer, where the dollars are in the receivable aging process. The key question is, "What percentage of my dollars are over 90 days? 120 days?" The next key question is, "What percentage of my dollars should be over 90 days? 120 days?" The first question will be answered through the *ATB*, the second will be subjected to a peer group and benchmark comparison.

The percent of dollars over 90 and 120 days is driven by the rule *that dollars having aged over 90 and 120 days are dollars that are in trouble*. Cleanly billed insurance dollars should be paid within 45 days as required by contract or regulation. Self-pay dollars should be collected at the time of service or, at most, 15 days after the first statement.

In Exhibit 1.4 the percentage over 90 days confirm our worst fears. Dollars are not being collected or worked effectively to get cash (how to effectively follow-up on insurance and self-pay collections will be discussed at length in Key Action Steps 5 and 6). "Our Practice's" staff needs to work older accounts, clean up claims and work with payers to expedite payment. The root causes of the aging dollars must be addressed to "stop the bleeding." The comparisons give us the needed information to determine that acceptable levels are not being met and better numbers are not only possible but required.

Exhibit 1.4 Percentage of dollars over 90 days

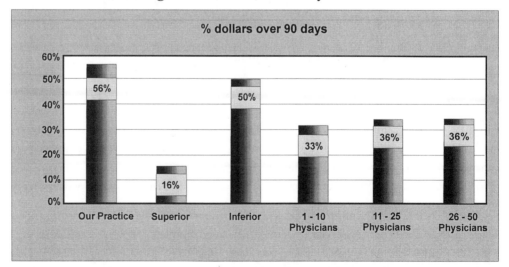

The percent of dollars over 120 days (Exhibit 1.5) further confirms that follow-up work is deficient (exacerbated perhaps by incomplete and inaccurate data collected at the front desk resulting in rejections) and remedies must be sought. If there had been a dramatic decrease from 90 days to 120 days, a case may have been made that follow-up was occurring or effectively, just not soon enough. However, with 49 percent of "Our Practice's" A/R dollars aged over 120 days, this argument is no longer possible.

Exhibit 1.5 Net days revenue outstanding

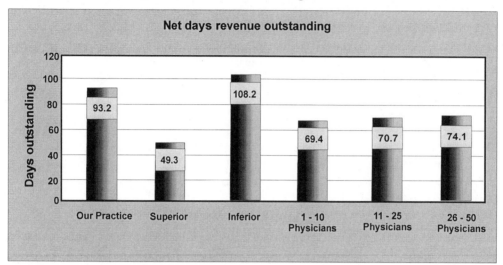

Payer breakdowns

The next level of analysis will be by payer, an objective statistic that will allow you to focus your efforts. It may be revealed only one or two major payers are slowing down your cash. However, an understanding of how your practice management system processes accounts is necessary.

> ▶ Does your system reclassify the self-pay portion after insurance payments to the self-pay financial class?

> ▶ Does your system reclassify supplemental insurance (secondary payers) to its financial class after the primary insurance?

> ▶ Are installment (budget plans) isolated from the self-pay financial class?

> ▶ Does your system re-age self-pay portions balances after insurance payments?

If your system does reclassify and re-age (and you have set up the system properly) then you will have a clear view of where your dollars are — if not, you will have to run additional reports to approximate the misallocated values.

A breakdown by major payer (or payer category) for NDRO and percentage of accounts over 90 days needs to be undertaken. Exhibit 1.6. is where we get an insight into what payers are disrupting cash flow. "Our Practice" is having severe problems with its self-pays, workers' compensation, Medicaid and contract commercial (managed care). In this analysis, the individual cash flow is revealed through each payer's NDRO calculation. This will focus the cash acceleration efforts (and resources) around payer-specific strategies.

Exhibit 1.6 Payer breakdown analysis

	Net A/R	Net A/R Mix	Net Revenue	Net Revenue Mix	Day's Revenue	NDRO
Blue Cross	$475,000	10%	$219,800	14%	$7,327	64.8
Commercial	$285,000	6%	$188,400	12%	$6,280	45.4
Contract - commercial	$665,000	14%	$188,400	12%	$6,280	105.9
Medicaid	$427,500	9%	$ 94,200	6%	$3,140	136.1
Medicare	$712,500	15%	$628,000	40%	$20,933	34.0
Workers' compensation	$712,500	15%	$ 78,500	5%	$2,617	272.3
Other	$47,500	1%	$ 15,700	1%	$523	90.8

Liquidation table

Another analytical tool is the "liquidation" table. In this table the payer mix (as represented by gross or net charges) is compared to the gross or net receivables (remember not to compare gross with net). This gives a quick look at the speed in which different payers make payment. If a payer represents 35 percent of your payer mix but represents only 20 percent of your receivables it indicates this payer — as compared to your other payers — liquidates cash at a faster pace than say, a payer who represents 20 percent of your payer mix but 40 percent of your receivables. Exhibit 1.7 provides insight into "Our Practice's" payers and how they compare to each other. This is an internal comparison and should be approached with some caution. That is, a particular payer may be an "excellent" payer when compared to other payers in your receivables, but an objective analysis may view it as only mediocre. However, it provides a snapshot and is useful in explaining to staff the state of "Our Practice's" receivables.

Exhibit 1.7 State of receivables

Payer	Percent of net charges	Percent of A/R	Liquidation rate
Blue Cross	14%	10%	Faster
Commercial	12%	6%	Faster
Contract - Commercial	12%	14%	Slower
Medicaid	6%	9%	Slower
Medicare	40%	15%	Faster
Workers' compensation	5%	15%	Slower
Other	1%	1%	Even
Self-pay	10%	30%	Slower

Bad debt

Your bad debt experience needs to be analyzed. A percentage of bad debt expense (write-off to bad debt less recoveries but does not include charity care) to gross revenue compared to national averages will provide a basis to see if your bad debt is too high or too low. Too high will indicate accounts are not being properly worked, too low may indicate you are allowing accounts to sit in your accounts receivable and may now be of no value. Accounts, as they age, lose their "collectability" due to: the patient moving out of the service area; the patient's economic situation changing for the worse; and the patient accruing newer debt which overrides your claim.

In Exhibit 1.8 "Our Practice," at 2.75 percent, is within range when compared to the 26-50 physician practice but certainly is not when compared to the 1-10 physician peer group. However, the major variables which impact bad debt — time-of-service collection effectiveness, statement cycle processing, account follow-up procedures, write-off procedures and collection agency collection effectiveness — must be analyzed to maximize their effectiveness and payback. Bad debt is an opportunity for each dollar retrieved from this category to fall right to the bottom line.

Exhibit 1.8 Bad debt expense composition

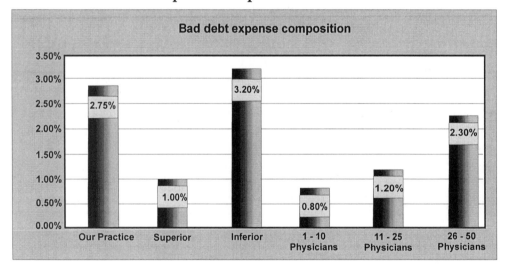

SUMMARY OF KEY ACTION STEP 1

► To improve cash flow and manage receivables, you need to monitor and analyse the key indicators.

► The key indicators will lead you to areas that need improvement and will be a necessary ingredient in goal setting and performance improvement initiatives.

► A receivables system needs to be managed and to manage you need accurate and timely data.

► When starting out on a cash acceleration or receivables performance improvement project, it is critical to lay down a baseline of the statistics discussed in this chapter.

► The effectiveness of any of your initiatives will show up in these statistics.

To Do List

Develop statistics, trend analysis, and comparisons for:

- ❑ Net charges and cash collections

- ❑ Net (or Gross) day's revenue outstanding

- ❑ Percent of dollars aged over 90 and 120 days

- ❑ Payer breakdowns

- ❑ Liquidation table

- ❑ Bad debt expense

Answer These Questions About "Our Practice":

- ❑ Do you have a "Cash Gap?"

- ❑ On what payers do you need to focus to have the maximum impact on cash?

- ❑ If you were to reduce your bad-debt expense by 1/2 percent, how many more dollars would that generate for your practice?

- ❑ How does your system reclassify self-pay accounts after insurance?

Key Action Step 2
IMPLEMENT PREREGISTRATION AND INSURANCE VERIFICATION SYSTEM

"Our Practice" is in trouble. The headache—introduced in Action Step 1—has subsided a bit after our statistical analysis. Using the analysis, discussions were held with staff who indicated a major source of the problems stemmed from inaccurate information being collected during the registration process. This resulted in managed care payers denying claims and rejecting billings for lack of referrals and pre-authorizations.

The most important functions, those which have the largest impact on cash collections, occur prior to the patient receiving service—this is where the *real* business office resides.

▶ **Preregistration function:** the collection of demographic, insurance and clinical information prior to the visit. This information will be reviewed for completeness and accuracy when the patient arrives for a visit. All information necessary for a complete registration should be collected prior to the patient arriving.

▶ **Insurance verification function:** the act of confirming a patient is indeed a subscriber of an insurance plan and eligible on that date of service. The subscriber's identification number and/or group number should also be verified for accuracy.

▶ **Insurance benefit levels determination function:** the act of determining the amount of money insurance will pay versus the amount the patient is expected to pay. It is critical at this point to determine if the deductible has been met, the service in question is covered, if there is a need for certifications and authorizations and if there is a copay or co-insurance.

▶ **Patient financial counselor function:** this is the art and science of working with the patient to review their financial options for payment on their bill. The options may include the use of credit cards, outside financing, budget (installment) plans or charity care. The financial counselor function is embedded in every function where financial matters are discussed with the patient. The person doing the scheduling, time-of-service registration or collection follow-up must be alert for problems involving the patient's inability to make timely payments. If your practice is large enough, specific staff members may be Patient Financial Counselors and patients would be referred to them. However, in most practices, this function will need to be a group effort, and all staff will need to be familiar with the Credit & Collection Policy and alternative financing options.

Benefits of preregistration and insurance verification

Patient service oriented

▶ At home, the patient is in a safe environment where financial and clinical information can be discussed confidentially and free from the stress of a medical visit.

▶ The patient, having attended to most of the paper work, will not have to endure a full registration at the visit and will be able to concentrate on their health.

▶ The patient will be informed of the financial expectations and alternative financing options of the practice. This information will allow the patient to make informed decisions about how they anticipate paying at the time of service.

Cash flow oriented

▶ Insurance verification process will identify any utilization review requirements of managed care organizations such as certifications and authorizations. It will also confirm the eligibility of the patient in the plan.

▶ Nothing disrupts cash flow worse than bad insurance and demographic information. The ability to collect and verify information before the visit is the stamp of a quality system and will shorten the payment cycle.

▶ Time-of-service cash collections will increase dramatically. A practice's self-pay cash payments (assuming an "average" payer mix) will range from 15-30 percent of total cash collected.

The steps in building a preregistration/insurance verification system

The preregistration and insurance verification processes are the cornerstones of a well-run receivables system. Without them your receivables statistics will never achieve (or exceed) the benchmark numbers. Because of the importance of the up front processes it is critical to develop and implement a preregistration, insurance verification, and time-of-service collections program as soon as possible (Time-of-service collections will be discussed in detail in chapter 3). Following is a list of activities for "Our Practice's" preregistration/insurance verification action plan:

▶ Review practice management software to determine data fields required and screen flows for input of demographic, insurance and clinical information.

▶ Review practice management software for *Insurance Master* module. An insurance master provides insurance plan benefits specific to major area employers. This will enable determination of benefit levels without making phone calls.

▶ Identify and document workflow and communication links between scheduling, preregistration, insurance verification, and financial counseling. Design the system to optimize information being available at the right time. By documenting the workflow, it will graphically highlight any gaps in the system. Identify current policies and procedures and update (or rewrite) to model previsit activities.

▶ Identify staffing needs to schedule, verify insurance, and determine benefit levels for 100 percent of all registrations. Subject your estimation of staffing to real life by taking ten scheduled visits and following procedure. Be aware of the times involved and the obstacles to efficient collection of information.

▶ Identify specific staff members. This may entail re-assigning personnel from back-end processes (account follow-up or lower payback functions).

▶ Train staff members in:

  ❏ Practice Management Software

    ❏ Scheduling

    ❏ Registration

    ❏ Patient accounting

  ❏ Required information and format needs by payers

  ❏ Credit & collection policy

  ❏ Alternative financing options

  ❏ Customer service

  ❏ Scripts for:

    ❏ Time-of-service payment discussions

    ❏ Insurance

    ❏ Alternative financing options

    ❏ Discussions with patients about delinquent accounts

▶ Coordinate activities of staff for scheduling/preregistration versus insurance verification work. The same person may accomplish this but, because of different information base (i.e., patient versus insurance company), it will require a two-step process.

▶ Communicate the importance of this process to physicians, other clinicians and business office staff.

▶ Develop a patient brochure that educates the patient on the benefits (to them) of the preregistration and insurance verification process, financial expectations of time-of-service payments, and alternative financing options.

▶ Implement and evaluate regularly.

Where the business office and point-of-service meet

The business office *is* preregistration and previsit insurance verification. The ability to set up an account transaction has more to do with successful receivable management than all the back-end processes combined. Patient financial counseling must occur prior to the visit when the patient is at their most open and responsive — not after billing. That the business office is working an account 30 days after service is an indication that the front-end processes have failed.

The back-office business office personnel are typically the knowledge base for all the different rules and requirements concerning managed care, Medicare, Medicaid, commercial and workers' compensation. They have a wealth of information on managed care contracts and their authorization and certification rules. The business office also has the unique perspective of seeing what procedures failed "upstream."

This information and knowledge needs to be brought forward in the process. Rather than fixing problems 30-90 days after service, any problems caused by inaccurate or incomplete information needs to be resolved prior to service.

When designing your system, determine when in the process staff should be doing follow-up activities. Remember these basic principles.

- ▶ The time spent doing self-pay follow-up collection calls will be better spent in doing financial counseling prior to service
- ▶ For the insurance follow-up staff will best spend their time confirming eligibility, ensuring billing requirements are complete and by ensuring the benefits levels are determined prior to service
- ▶ Always strive to place the activities as early in the process as possible.

The traits of a quality preregistration/insurance verification program

- ▶ Staff understands, appreciates and effectively communicates the financial expectations of the practice.
- ▶ Efficient and accurate collection of vital information required for future communication (such as correct spelling of names, complete addresses and telephone numbers, as well as insurance companies and insurance identification numbers)
- ▶ Very few denials for lack of pre-authorization through insurance verification
- ▶ Low denial rate of reinbursement level due to thorough advance checking of applicable benefit levels
- ▶ Cash acceleration due to high collection rate of patient portion at time of service
- ▶ Effective identification of patients presenting credit risk
- ▶ Use of credit cards

The patient financial counseling function

Patient financial counseling begins with the first patient contact. This function, combined with time-of-service collections and a tight statement cycle (see chapter 7) are the three activities, which will dramatically reduce "Our Practice's" bad debt expense.

The ability for staff members to be successful in finding the right option for the patient depends on the mix and variety of options made available by the practice. The base menu of *alternative financing options* is:

➤ Credit cards

➤ Outside financing source (i.e. bank loan)

➤ Payment (installment) plans

➤ Charity care

Credit cards

The use of credit cards is an excellent alternative financing option for both the practice and the patient. The practice receives cash immediately and the patients have a financing vehicle allowing them to make monthly payments based on their financial situation. The patient is fully in control of how they wish to conduct their financial affairs and will pay a premium (interest on unpaid balances) if they need to exercise credit.

The use of credit cards needs to be sold to the patients. Preregistration discussions with the patient should include this option for time-of-service payment. Other techniques for selling the programs are:

➤ Signs at the point-of-service. Make sure the patient is aware of what credit cards "Our Practice" accepts.

➤ Print the credit card option on patient statements.

➤ Remind staff to "push" this option when counseling patients who are having difficulty making payments.

Outside financing

Setting up outside financing for a patient is more cumbersome than credit cards but is an effective means for larger dollar balances. These loans are written as "full recourse," which means if the patient defaults, the bank will demand payment from the clinic on the full amount of the unpaid balance. It then is up to the clinic to collect the balance from the patient. Even as "no risk" loans, most financial institutions do not wish to be bothered with these lower balance programs. However, the financial institution that currently has the practice's business should be approached.

As with credit cards, the benefit for the practice is that it receives cash and removes itself from the financing business. A basic procedural model would be:

➤ Patient agrees to this arrangement

➤ Bank credit application is filled out by patient and clinic staff

- A promissory note (agreement to pay with amounts and effective interest rates) is signed
- Bank pays practice
- Patient pays bank principle and interest
- In case of default, bank demands amount of unpaid balance (and unpaid interest) from practice.

Payment plans

Payment plans, also called installment plans, is not the option of choice. In effect, payment plans turn the practice into a financing company while adding cost to the practice through additional statement processing and follow-up. This option should be used judiciously.

Payment terms should never be extended beyond three monthly payments. The initial payment needs to be received immediately (or within five days) to substantiate a level of sincerity.

Charity care

Charity care is a financing option. Not a good one—but an option. It is useful for those rare instances where the patient is clearly unable to pay and will not be experiencing an upturn in their fortunes anytime soon. The charity care program needs to be outlined in the practice's credit and collection policy. If a charity care program is not offered, that should be noted in the credit and collection policy. Authorization approvals for charity care should be granted by the practice administrator or patient's physician. Charity care dollars granted should be reported on financial statements.

SUMMARY OF KEY ACTION STEP 2

▶ Preregistration and insurance verification *is* the business office, enhancing registration accuracy and cash flow.

▶ Insurance verification reduces claim denials and rejections dramatically.

▶ Insurance verification of benefit level is necessary for time-of-service collections.

▶ Preregistration will reduce substantially bad-debt expense through early identification of credit risk and providing patient financial counseling on options for payment.

▶ Helps in collecting former bad debts or resolving present problems.

▶ Patient service is heightened through providing information to patients for their personal financial decision making.

To Do List

☐ Research your practice management system to determine if there is an insurance/employer master.

☐ Develop a credit and collection policy which emphasizes time-of-service collections.

☐ Train scheduling personnel to educate the patient that payment is expected at time of service.

☐ At time of scheduling, have staff do a full preregistration by collecting all demographic and insurance information.

☐ Train staff on calling insurance for verification of eligibility and benefit levels.

☐ Design patient brochure explaining policy of practice and the process.

Answer These Questions About "Our Practice":

☐ What is the denial rate for lack of precertifications or "...not eligible on date of service"?

☐ What is rejection rate for claims submitted to insurance companies containing incorrect information?

☐ What are the reasons for the rejections?

☐ Do you inform patients prior to service that you expect payment at time of service?

☐ Do the back-end collection processes hurt or help customer service? How necessary are they?

Key Action Step 3
PUT IN PLACE A HIGH PERFORMANCE TIME-OF-SERVICE PAYMENT PROGRAM

If you have put in place an effective preregistration/insurance verification program then a collection at the time-of-service program is already 99 percent complete. At the time of the patient visit (or even prior to the visit), the patient will be aware of your payment policy and the amount of their expected payment. It will be the mere act of asking, "Will you be paying by cash, credit card or check?" to complete the process.

Time-of-service collection is a critical component in the financial success of "Our Practice." The benefits are:

► Expedites cash flow from patient portion by an average of 60 days
► Lowers bad-debt expense through effective financial counseling, credit risk management, and, if necessary, early collection agency placement
► Heightens productivity through reduced self-pay collection follow-up
► Lowers cost through reduced statement processing
► Identifies patients truly in need of charity care alternative financial options
► Fulfills utilization requirements of managed care contracts
► Deductibles, copayments and co-insurance are designed to remind patient that healthcare is not free.

The psychological advantage

A person's thinking about health care payments changes radically the moment they leave the practice without paying their bill. Before service and at the point of service, their health is the number one priority in their life and they have the mindset of a patient. They are motivated to make payment because they are motivated to restore their health.

When they leave the practice, they are no longer a patient—they are now a "debtor." They revert back to being an economic animal with obligations to many different creditors: mortgage payments, credit card payments, utility bills and their children's education needs. Your bill will begin competing with all other bills, and, if the patient's (debtor's) financial situation is tight. "Our Practice's" bill will always come in last.

Do not lose the psychological advantage. Ask for payment when the patient is most motivated to pay. (See Exhibit 3.1)

Exhibit 3.1 Differences in patient's vs. debtor priorities

Patient Priorities	Debtor Priorities
☐ Health care	☐ Home
☐ Home	☐ Car loan
☐ Car loan	☐ Utilities
☐ Utilities	☐ Bank loan
☐ Bank loan	☐ Credit cards
☐ Credit cards	☐ Insurance premiums
☐ Insurance premiums	☐ Health care

The largest obstacle to implementing time-of-service collections: staff concerns

Effective time-of-service collection programs are all about attitude—to be effective your staff has to believe in and sell the program. Many times programs fizzle because the staff is just too uncomfortable with the idea of asking someone for money. Therefore, take the time to facilitate meeting(s) with your staff to discuss their concerns and to help them develop their collection skills.

Concerns which you may encounter — and a response:

"Asking people for money is bad customer service."

Surprising people by asking for money — without informing them of your expectation of payment at the time of service — *is* bad customer service. But in the preregistration process you have set the stage for them to *expect* you to ask them for payment. Any objections have already been overcome. Giving people information to make informed decisions about their financial obligations is great customer service.

"I feel uncomfortable asking people for money. It seems rude."

Staff needs to be trained in the art of asking for payment. In every other financial transaction of your patient's life they expect to make payment (or arrange for payment) at the point of sale. Staff needs to understand the patient will not be offended and their fears of the "hostile" patient are unfounded. Have the staff, as a group, write scripts responding to their worst fears. Have them act out the scripts until they feel comfortable. Some staff will be more comfortable (and better) than others in asking for payment. Rotate staff to see who can get the highest collections. Ask the top performers to share their secrets to success with the others.

"I feel uncomfortable handling money. If it gets lost, I'll be blamed."

Explain to staff there are accounting procedures to ensure cash is reconciled. These procedures protect the people who handle cash from being accused unfairly of losing or stealing the money. Show them the cash receipts process.

The second largest obstacle to implementing time-of-service collections: dealing with co-insurance

Where many practices turn faint of heart and decide not to pursue a time-of-service collections program is the inability to estimate patient charges. In the case of copays and deductibles this is not a problem since these are fixed amounts (however, you may need to contact insurer to determine if deductible has been met). It is when we get into the area of co-insurance — where the patient liability is a percent of charges — that complications arise.

The best approach for estimating the patient's portion of the bill is to calculate the exact amount of charges from the encounter form (a.k.a. superbill). From the encounter form, the checked services can be summed for an exact amount. This will, however, take coordination of activities between the front desk and the physician:

▶ Because the payment will be made *after* service and not before, the patient will need to be routed back to the reception or cashier area.

▶ The physicians will have to fill out the encounter charges in "real time" so as not to delay the patient or undermine the payment process.

▶ If the physician will be waiting for test results to determine a diagnosis, the encounter form will need to be routed back to the physician for completion.

If there is a high variability of charges based on individual patient's needs (i.e., an in-office surgical procedure) you may need to rely on an estimate of charges based on past experience. An analysis of International Classification of Diseases, Ninth Revision (ICD-9) procedure code by physician will provide a solid approximation of charges. It will not be exact and either a balance bill or a refund check will need to be sent.

Helpful reminders—signs and brochures

You can't say it too often or in too many different ways. Discrete signs indicating payment is expected at the time of service should be displayed at the reception and cashier areas. If, under your managed care contracts, the practice is obligated to collect copayments and deductibles at the time of service, this very helpful information should be displayed.

Brochures, which describe the financial expectations for the patient, should be developed. It should include information for the patients who are under financial duress and would like financial counseling as well. The brochure can be effectively used in the financial counseling interview process to walk the patient through the policies of the practice and provides them with a document for future reference.

Having the patient sign an acceptance of the financial policy further enhances a patient's understanding of the practice's financial expectations.

Goal setting

The utopian ideal for time-of-service collections is 100 percent of all payments for noninsured self-pay balances and insured patient's copayments, deductibles, and co-insurance. However, the first step in the process is to establish a current experience as a baseline for improvement. If your current experience is 10 percent collection of noninsured balances and 30 percent of co-pay collections, it is unreasonable to expect 90 percent effectiveness next week. In this case, set interim goals leading up to the final goal of 100 percent.

Working with high credit risk patients

There will always be patients who present special problems. Despite your best efforts at patient counseling before service, some patients will appear who are not prepared to pay. Because of "Our Practice's" effective preregistration program, the number of patients filling this category will diminish — but they will still exist nonetheless.

If they are a consistent problem and appear at the "Our Practice" with prior accounts unpaid, it is time to do some financial counseling.

- ▶ Find a confidential area where you can talk to the patient.
- ▶ Explain to the patient the policy of "Our Practice" and ask them what special circumstances they are under which prevent them from paying their accounts.
- ▶ Listen to their concerns. Only three percent of patients who do not pay are true delinquents — the other 97 percent have good intentions but need help in their personal finances.
- ▶ As the patient explains their financial situation you may see opportunities which could aid the patient in fulfilling their obligation.
- ▶ Be prepared with the alternative financing options to fit their unique situation.

The base options required, in the order of benefit to the practice, are (See Key Action Step 1 for detailed explanation):

- ▶ Credit cards
- ▶ Outside financing source (i.e., bank loan for high dollar balances)
- ▶ Payment (installment) plans
- ▶ Charity care

In the financial counselor role, you are providing information to the patient so they are better able to make decisions. It is your job to overcome any obstacles to payment and — before the patient leaves — get a commitment (time of payment and amount).

If after an examination of their financial status it is determined they are able to pay but refuse, or are habitual credit delinquents, then you may come to the conclusion they need to seek services elsewhere. In the credit and collection policy, address the conditions under which a patient would be terminated. The termination policy should outline procedures for notification, time periods, and exclusions for emergency services.

For those patients who forget their credit card

For those well-meaning patients who forgot to bring their credit card, checkbook or any cash there is a technique your staff needs to implement. Give the patient a form which indicates the amount owed and the payment method (check or credit card). Also, include a self-addressed stamped envelope. Request as soon as the patient returns home, they fill in the credit card information (or make out a check), put it in the envelope and mail it back today. This way you are making payment easy for the patient while underlining the commitment to payment at the time of service. Hopefully, they won't forget their credit card or checkbook next time.

SUMMARY OF KEY ACTION STEP 3

▶ **Time-of-service collection is critical to cash flow and lowering bad debt expense.**

▶ **Time-of-service collections enhances patient service.**

▶ **The preregistration and insurance verification programs must be in place for an effective time-of-service program.**

▶ **Patient financial counseling starts at scheduling.**

▶ **Train your staff to be comfortable with requesting payment.**

▶ **Make it easy for your patients to pay with credit cards.**

▶ **Have a full menu of financial options.**

To Do List

❑ Train your staff in feeling comfortable requesting payment.

❑ Identify services where you need to estimate charges for co-insurance situations.

❑ Have signs reminding patients on the expectation of payment at time of service.

Answer These Questions About "Our Practice":

❑ What is your collection rate at the time of service?

❑ What should your collection rate be at the time of service?

❑ Is your staff open to requesting payments?

Key Action Step 4
PROTECT AND ENHANCE YOUR REVENUE

It's running as smooth as clockwork. The patient was preregistered and counseled on the expectation of payment at the time of service. "Our Practice" called the patient's managed care firm or other insurer and verified they are a subscriber in good standing, the services were covered, and there would be a $15.00 co-payment. The patient arrived right on schedule and the smiling receptionist reviewed all the demographic and insurance information for accuracy and then requested and received the $15.00 co-payment. The patient decided to pay by credit card. The patient is ushered immediately in to see the doctor.

In terms of the revenue cycle, we are at the charge generation and coding stage. Charge generation and coding — the revenue cycle activities which document services rendered — decides the amount of money "Our Practice" will bill and the amount of money the payer will decide to pay. Sloppy controls at this phase will result in lost dollars from no charges being generated, dollars held up due to slow processing, underpayments (or overpayments) due to incorrect coding, and possible sanctions due to out-of-compliance coding.

To ensure optimum (rightful) reimbursement, procedures and controls must:

- ▶ Capture 100 percent of all services and supplies rendered and documented
- ▶ Accurately identify and code the appropriate level of service
- ▶ Accurately identify and code the diagnosis
- ▶ Input information within one day of service for timely billing

The missing ticket report

A missing ticket report (MTR) is a management report identifying encounters without accompanying charges. This may be due to the physician holding the encounter form, a patient inadvertently leaving the practice with the encounter form, backlogs in data entry, a canceled encounter or because the encounter form is lost. In any of these situations, it is costing the practice money.

Physicians are key in this process. A policy describing physician behaviors (written, endorsed, and supported by the physicians) in filing complete and accurate encounter forms within one day of service needs to be in place and enforced.

There are two MTR systems which must be employed: scheduled office encounters and hospital encounters. The scheduled office encounter is the simpler system. The hospital encounter will need to be designed to meet your individual practice and hospital(s) resources.

Scheduled office encounters

All mainstream practice management systems employ some form of a missing ticket report. The system allows for "on-demand" reports to be run which will detail all the scheduled encounters that are missing charge information.

The MTR should be run daily. All cancelled visits need to be deleted, physicians need to be contacted to determine where encounter forms are and data entry needs to be monitored to ensure they are at zero backlog.

If you do not have automated system capabilities, use a manual log system to verify that all scheduled visits have been billed.

Hospital encounters

It is here that you will have to be innovative. The design of your MTR for hospital encounters will be based on the resources and cooperation of the hospital(s) and the organizational and communication skills of your physicians. Following is a model MTR system for hospitals:

➤ The hospital(s) fax or mail their registration "front sheet" notifying the practice of all the practice's patients who have been admitted to the hospital. The front sheet will include admitting diagnosis, room number, time and date of admission.

➤ Your physicians supply you with their schedule of the next day's hospital visits by patient.

➤ Physicians submit their encounter forms one day following service; or,

➤ The hospital(s) places, inside the patient's hospital chart, your encounter forms. When completed, the hospital mails encounter forms to "Our Practice."

➤ A log system reconciles the physicians' schedule and the hospital notifications with charges.

It is probable not all of the above control functions will be available. Maybe your hospitals will not be as accommodating or your physicians as organized. However, it is critical that a control system is built to ensure hospital charges are not lost.

The importance of the encounter form

The encounter form (a.k.a. superbill or routing slip) is an important form that aids in ensuring all services are accounted for (and billed) and coding complexities are simplified. In effect, the encounter form is a reflection of your practice. It identifies clearly and precisely the evaluation and management (E&M) codes, your most ordered services and supplies (with current procedural terminology (CPT-4 designation), and your most used ICD-9 diagnosis codes. This does not mean trying to jam all the services and ICD-9s your practice has ever used — only those most commonly used.

It is a good idea to run reports analyzing what ICD-9s and CPT-4s predominate in your practice. Segregate the resulting CPT-4 services into logical groupings (i.e., lab services versus injections versus E&M codes). Design the bill for ease of use featuring quick identification of procedures and diagnoses.

Coding and the physician

Coding is the responsibility of the physician. Incorrect coding which does not conform to government compliance will ultimately have to be answered by the physician. While a practice may aid the physician with staff who code (hopefully they are certified), it is still the physician who must review the final codes for accuracy.

Because of the fear of overcoding, undercoding is far more prevalent. This means dollars, which are rightfully due the practice, are being lost. This is an area that has significant opportunity for revenue enhancement without additional resource consumption.

It is recommended an annual audit of your physicians' coding is undertaken to ensure no over or undercoding is taking place. The audit results will probably indicate a need for a corrective action which will include additional and periodic training for physicians and staff.

The problem of no-shows

Patients who miss appointments disrupt a practice and result in lost revenue. It is important to develop a no-show policy which include penalties and patient notifications. The policy should be communicated to all new patients, re-addressed in the scheduling process and included in the patient brochure.

Each initial no-show should get a letter informing them of the practice's policy, why keeping appointments is a courtesy to other patients and, if it occurs again, a service fee would be charged. If it does happen again, the service fee would be assessed and would have to be paid prior to scheduling another visit. If the patient does not pay they would be barred from further service. Upon the third no-show, they have established themselves as a chronic "no-shower." It doesn't mean they are a bad person, just someone who has trouble keeping commitments. However, at this point, the service fee would be charged prior to the service asking for a monetary commitment to reserving a visit.

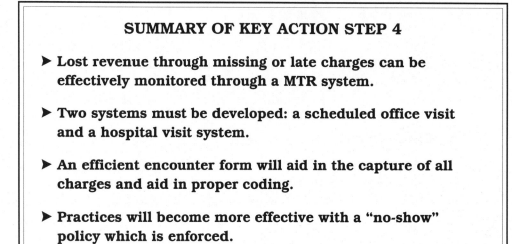

SUMMARY OF KEY ACTION STEP 4

➤ Lost revenue through missing or late charges can be effectively monitored through a MTR system.

➤ Two systems must be developed: a scheduled office visit and a hospital visit system.

➤ An efficient encounter form will aid in the capture of all charges and aid in proper coding.

➤ Practices will become more effective with a "no-show" policy which is enforced.

To Do List

❑ **Run MTR on daily basis.**

❑ **Identify missing and late charges, assess status charges and capture them for billing.**

❑ **Review encounter forms. Assess whether "Our Practice's" diagnosis and services are displayed.**

❑ **Audit coding for under or overcoding.**

❑ **Develop a no-show policy**

Answer These Questions About "Our Practice":

❑ **What is the average number of days from time of service to charge entry into billing system?**

❑ **What are the reasons for the number of days over two days from time of service to charge entry?**

❑ **What charges are currently "lost?"**

❑ **Are your physicians actively involved in the coding process?**

❑ **If staff performs coding, are they certified? When was the last time they went to a seminar on coding?**

❑ **When was the last coding audit conducted?**

Key Action Step 5
IMPLEMENT A "CLEAN" CLAIM AND AGGRESSIVE INSURANCE FOLLOW-UP PROGRAM

Cash from insurance carriers will represent, based on specialty and demographics of your service area, 65-90 percent of your total practice cash flow. It is critical insurance claim processing is effective (accurate) and efficient (automated). If "Our Practice" is able to create a "clean" claim, payment will be forthcoming without further resources expended (barring any payer problems).

The billing process is fully dependent on all the processes that go before it. In simple terms, billing is merely the processing, coordination and cataloguing of demographic, insurance, charge and coding information onto a HCFA 1500 form. Processing, coordination and cataloguing are the domain of your automated practice management system.

This chapter will focus on the processes necessary to create a "clean" insurance claim and collection techniques to prompt faster payments from the insurance carriers.

The "unclean" claim

Payer rejections occur when claims are filed with incorrect or inaccurate information. The reason for payer-specific rejections must be reviewed on a monthly basis at a minimum. The most common insurance rejections are:

- ▶ Subscriber number is missing or incorrect
- ▶ Plan or group number is missing or inaccurate
- ▶ ICD-9 diagnosis codes are missing
- ▶ ICD-9 diagnosis codes do not support the services and procedures given
- ▶ Incorrect or missing dates
- ▶ Same day, multiple visits are billed without explanation
- ▶ Supporting documentation missing

Analyze the rejections and denials. Prioritize by dollar impact on your cash. Choose the highest priority item and develop a strategy to correct the problem.

When you have resolved that issue, proceed to the next. Do not try to solve all the problems at once.

Analysis of your "product"

Billing is a quantifiable art. In Exhibit 5.1 we see that "Our Practice" has a problem with specific insurance carriers. Contract commercial (105.9 NDRO), Medicaid (136.1 NDRO) and workers' compensation (272.3 NDRO) are payers which are certainly not performing well.

Exhibit 5.1 Insurance carrier analysis

	Net A/R	Net A/R Mix	Net Revenue	Net Revenue Mix	Days' Revenue	NDRO
Blue Cross	$475,000	14%	$219,800	16%	$ 7,327	64.8
Commercial	$285,000	9%	$188,400	13%	$ 6,280	45.4
Contract -Commercial	$665,000	20%	$188,400	13%	$ 6,280	105.9
Medicaid	$427,500	13%	$ 94,200	7%	$ 3,140	136.1
Medicare	$712,500	21%	$628,000	44%	$20,933	34.0
Worker's Compensation	$712,500	21%	$ 78,500	6%	$ 2,617	272.3
Other	$ 47,500	1%	$ 15,700	1%	$ 523	90.8

These payers are destroying the practice's cash flow. In the case of Contract-Commercial, assuming payment should be received in 45 days, the cash that is removed from the cash flow approximates $382,000!

Each Day's Net Revenue (potential cash)	$6,280
Net Day's Revenue Outstanding — Current	105.9
Net Day's Revenue Outstanding — Goal	45.0
Net Day's Revenue Outstanding — Opportunity (105.9 - 45)	60.9
Cash Opportunity (60.9 * $6,280)	$382,452

Reporting on payment and rejection analysis

A payment and rejection analysis with special emphasis on contract-commercial, Medicaid and workers' compensation needs to be undertaken. This will be an audit with a quality assessment of your claims processing "product." It will reveal how long processes are taking (time from service to bill, time of bill to time of payment) and the reasons for claim payment delays.

In Exhibit 5.2 the payment and rejection analysis for Contract-Commercial indicates that "Our Practice" is having a real problem with the plans' group number identification. It is probable the up front personnel are unaware of the importance of this key bit of information.

Exhibit 5.2 Commercial insurance

Account number	Billed amount	Date					Rejection reasons — Dollars held			
		Service	Service to Bill (in days)	Bill	Bill to payment (in days)	Payment	Group number	No coverage	I.D. Sub-scriber	Other
1234567	$ 137	1/20/00	2	1/22/00	45	5/07/00			137	
1234624	2,100	1/22/00	11	2/02//00	36	3/09/00	2100			
1234663	158	1/24/00	98	5/01/00	44	6/14/00		345		
1234702	345	1/26/00	3	1/29/00	39	3/08/00				
1234741	189	1/28/00	23	2/20/00	41	4/01/00	189			
1234780	67	1/30/00	27	2/26/00	65	5/01/00				67
1234819	89	2/01/00	24	2/25/00	43	4/08/00			89	
1234858	198	1/03/00	30	3/04/00	29	4/02/00				
1234897	212	2/05/00	22	2/27/00	102	6/08/00				
1234936	1,500	2/07/00	37	3/15/00	56	5/10/00	1500			
1234975	378	1/09/00	22	3/02/00	45	4/16/00			378	
1235014	220	2/11/00	17	2/28/00	44	4/12/00				
1235053	120	2/13/00	14	2/27/00	50	4/17/00			120	
1235092	67	2/15/00	18	3/04/00	67	5/10/00				67
1235131	78	2/17/00	76	5/03/00	43	6/15/00				
1235270	67	2/19/00	2	2/21/00	56	4/17/00				67
1235209	135	2/21/00	38	3/30/00	54	5/23/00	135			
1235248	235	2/23/00	30	3/24/00	34	4/27/00				
1235287	768	2/25/00	50	4/15/00	23	5/08/00	768			
1235326	67	2/27/00	80	5/17/00	87	8/12/00				67
1235365	156	2/29/00	28	3/28/00	44	5/11/00				
	$7,286		31.05		49.86		4692	345	724	268

The steps in the audit process are:

► Pick a random sample of accounts that have been paid. The sample size should be no less than 20 for each payer category. The payer category should represent a significant payer group whether a financial class (i.e., workers' compensation) or an individual plan (Aetna).

► For each payer, do a system "look-up" of the account. Record date of service, date of bill and date of payment. Also identify reasons for re-bills or follow-up calls. Hopefully, your staff is doing a good job of posting payments, memos and rejection information to the system. If not, you will be forced to cross-reference to the payer's Explanation of Benefit (EOB).

► Summarize findings

► Develop an action plan to correct the problem. It looks like "Our Practice" needs to retrain staff on collection of group plan numbers at preregistration, verification of number at insurance verification and confirmation at the time of visit through a review of the patient's insurance card. It also appears to produce a "clean claim," with rework and rebills taking an average of 31.05 days.

The prebill edits

Prebill edits are data field requirements in your automated system which demand either that a value is present and/or the value is in a payer required form. (As an example: the group number may demand a specific plan prefix.) The complexities in trying to remember payer claims' requirements mandates "Our Practice" to maximize its automated system to stop claims from being billed which will be sent back as "rejected."

By stopping an unclean claim from billing, it will expedite cash by the amount of time it would have taken to receive a rejection, clean it up and then reprocess for payment. Your system prebill edits need to be set as tightly as the payers' edits.

Rejection reports or online edits need to be reviewed and worked daily. It is, in effect, an on-going payment and rejection analysis. A manager needs to review these reports to ensure retraining is performed and performance improvement strategies are developed and implemented.

Electronic claims submission (ECS)

The filing of claims electronically is a must. Electronic claim filing is the creation of a computer file which contains the data necessary to complete a HCFA 1500. The file is either directly submitted via modem, internet connection, tape, disk or "downloaded" to a personal computer (PC). In the download system, a prebill editor, or "scrubber," will check the claim against the payer edits. If the claim is "clean," it will then be submitted.

Any practice with a significant claim volume must take advantage of ECS technology if it aspires to maximizing cash flow and minimizing costs. Benefits of ECS include:

► **Faster payment than paper claims.** The payers' process ECSs on set schedules and processing is not delayed by manual processing complications (i.e., understaffing, sickness, vacation and holidays).

► **Cleaner claims.** Most payer systems will have an edit check in the submission process. Claims failing this check will be "suspended" waiting immediate correction. Manual claim checks will be sent back in 30-60 days.

► **Reduced cost.** The amount of labor which goes into a paper claim evaporates, as well as the supplies and postage expense.

► **Quality and consistency of data.** ECS demands process protocols be respected. As pre-edits and payer edit systems provide information about out-of-range data, the quality and consistency of data will improve.

► **Better management control.** Through ECS management reports, managers are advised of the billing status of the claim and verify the claims were received. The payers' edit reports will also give instant management feedback.

Payer specific strategies

Each payer is unique and unique strategies will need to be implemented to overcome billing obstacles. Following are billing ideas on specific payers:

► **Workers' compensation.** It is always a challenge. It is critical to ascertain the patient's employer, the employer's workers' compensation carrier and the supporting documentation the carrier requires. When a patient indicates the injury or condition is work-related, the alarms should go off. Time needs to be spent verifying that the employer agrees the injury or condition is work related, the carrier has received the claim and has all the supporting documentation to approve payment.

► **Medicare.** This is your fastest payer. Make sure your claim is clean and your coding has been reviewed for accuracy. If you can get this claim in on the day of service, you will be receiving payment within three weeks.

► **Medicaid.** If you are able to generate a clean claim, this can be one of your faster payers yet probably one of your worst in terms of level of reimbursement.

► **Commercial.** Each insurer will have to be dealt with separately. Based on their internal systems competency, they can be one of your faster and better payers. For insurers with poor claim processing capabilities, effective and timely follow-up will be a must.

► **Health Maintenance Organizations (HMO) and Preferred Provider Organizations (PPO).** Utilization guidelines (referrals and authorizations) make HMOs more complicated to work with. Make sure all personnel in the revenue cycle are aware of the contract requirements.

► **Preferred Provider Organizations (PPO).** PPOs make things difficult because they add a third party into the payer and provider relationship. The PPO, in effect, is a contract negotiator and claim repricer. For PPOs you will need to ensure not only the PPO received the claim but also the payer received the claim from the PPO.

To effectively plot out unique strategies for each payer, it is critical *a Third Party Fact Sheet* for each payer is established. The fact sheet will:

➤ Identify important contact personnel

➤ Define the hierarchy of authorities for approving claim payments

➤ Detail the sequence of claim processing steps

➤ Delineate authorization requirements

➤ Outline referral requirements

➤ Provide supporting documentation for specific services

➤ Document unique billing requirements

➤ Provide a history of major reasons for payment denials and rejections

Insurance collection follow-up

Despite "Our Practice's" best efforts, there will always be insurance claims which, for many reasons, will not be paid unless staff dedicated to collection follow-up intervene. The major reasons given for non-paid accounts are:

➤ No claim received

➤ Waiting for information from patient

➤ Coverage under other insurance

➤ Work-related injury or condition

➤ Third-party liability

➤ "Pending" for medical review or preexisting condition

➤ Subject to deductible

➤ Paid directly to patient

➤ Unable to identify subscriber

A key element in the collection follow-up process is the processing of correspondence/mail received from the payers concerning claim filings. These informational missives are a gold mine of information and need to be worked daily. They will inform you about deductibles, information requests sent to the patient and denials.

Another key is that staff needs to be dedicated to this function. It is not sufficient to ask certain staff members to try to "fit in" collection follow-up with their other activities. The "other activities" will always win out. If you are unable to dedicate a full position to this function, dedicate a specific staff member for a specific amount of time at specific times during the week.

The "DOC" approach to collections

The DOC approach is a sequence of three events which, when done effectively, will result in "winning" on 100 percent of the accounts called. The underlying concept is you're making follow-up calls to persuade the payer into action not merely to memo information received.

> ➤ **Decision maker.** Get to the decision maker even if that means the president of the insurance company. Staff should not waste their time arguing with claims "clerks" who are only able to tell you "I'm sorry the claim is pending."

> ➤ **Overcome the obstacles.** Your collectors need to be innovative thinkers who like a good competition. When presented with obstacles to claim payment they need to be one step ahead of the payer. They need the resources to provide additional documentation and access to coding personnel (physicians).

> ➤ **Commitment.** On every call a commitment needs to be reached. If the payer needs more information, an agreement specifying when (and how) they will receive information needs to be forged. If they have agreed payment is forthcoming, the amount and when can be expected needs to be reached and noted in your files.

There will be times when you are stymied. Perhaps the payer refuses or seems unable pay. It is then you must bring in your biggest and best weapon — the patient. If you are dealing with an HMO, they will tell you, per the contract, you are not able to talk to the patient about the claim. This is not true. You have every right in the world to work with *your patient* in resolving *problems* with *their insurance*. Also, indicate to the HMO, per the contract, they were to have paid you 15 (or 30 or 45) days ago.

Before communicating with the patient, tell the payer's decision maker that you are forced into calling the patient. Also get the decision maker's name, title and phone number. Explain to the payer you will be asking the patient to call them so the payer can explain to the patient why their insurance company is not paying bills for services covered under their contract.

When you talk to the patient, make sure they know you are on their side. The patient is paying their premiums, the physician is providing a covered service, but the payer is not holding up their end of the bargain. Ask the patient if they wouldn't mind calling the decision maker. Also request them to call you back to tell you what occurred and if they need any further assistance.

Educate your follow-up staff on the "DOC" approach and make sure you provide them with the necessary authority to overcome the obstacles.

Collection effectiveness

Collection success is about cash receipts and should not be confused with merely gathering information (i.e., claim's representative says "claim pending no payment date set"). Reviewing accounts aged over 60 days should be done on a regular basis.

A formal study of collection effectiveness is called a "payment history analysis." Randomly select ten accounts for each member of the collection staff. Review each account to determine:

▶ When the collection follow-up started

▶ If the collector was persistent in getting at the decision maker

▶ If there were multiple "rebills"noted without agreement

▶ If insurance contacts were noted with title and phone number

▶ If collector overcame the obstacles

▶ If claims were resolved with promise for payment for a specific date

▶ If collector was aggressive enough — persistent enough

▶ If there was too much follow-up activity on a consistent basis (This is a sign contact is not effective. The collector probably needs additional training in closing the account.)

▶ If payment promises are monitored (Calls need to be made on the date, or day after, if payment was not received as promised.)

▶ If collector is getting agreement on payment or an alternative course of action

▶ If there is a specific, clear and understandable agreement

▶ If the collector memos the system effectively and efficiently

The reviews need to be shared with the individual collector. Common obstacles experienced by collection staff should be quantified and discussed at team meetings.

Bring in the payer representative

Sometimes a payer's ability to process a claim is such a mess that you will need to work the accounts as a group. Again, you will need to get the attention of a decision maker — probably an "account representative."

Bring them into your facility and provide them with a summary aging analysis derived from your aged trial balance. Explain to them the total cash impact caused by their delinquency in making payment.

In the initial meeting the payer needs to explain to you why they are unable to make payments per the contract. If the reason is because of their internal systems, the discussion needs to center around a prepayment plan in the amount of the delinquency to be refunded when their system is functioning.

If the reason(s) for nonpayment are other than a payer system failure, the meeting must generate a plan of action; that is, what do you and the payer need to do to be in compliance with the overriding contractual agreement. Make sure this meeting does not become confrontational — they need you and you need them. Again, "overcome the obstacles."

Before the meeting ends, reach an agreement on the actions to be taken. After the meeting, be persistent; keep up your end of the agreement and insist they do the same.

Goal setting and documentation

To be successful in running an efficient and effective follow-up collection function, goals need to be set, monitored and rewarded — both individually and as a group. People enjoy being successful. Successes are impossible without quantifiable or observable targets.

Establish a goal for each collector to resolve at least 45 accounts per eight-hour period. Identify the largest dollar balances and set a cash dollar amount to accompany the number of resolved accounts. Project this amount out for a monthly collector goal and summarize it for a total group goal.

Have each collector fill out a *Collection Action Report* daily, as shown in Exhibit 5.3. This report is crucial in establishing that the collector reached an agreement with the payer that will ultimately result in payment. This report establishes that the goals are being met and the staff understands the DOC approach to account resolution.

Exhibit 5.5   Collection action report

Step 1: Get to the **D**ecision Maker

Step 2: **O**vercome the Obstacles

Step 3: Get the $ Commitment

Account #	$ Promised	Date promised	If no $ commitment — What action have you taken?	Follow-up date

Total $ Promised: _____   For the _____ day of _____. Page _____ of _____.

Review the reports in short, weekly meetings. These meetings are a tremendous forum for discussing payer specific problems and discussing account resolution techniques. Make sure when goals are reached, they are appropriately celebrated and incentives are distributed. This discussion will be expanded in the Key Action Step 12 "The Implementation Plan And Motivation For Results."

SUMMARY OF KEY ACTION STEP 5

► **Your major cash stream comes from insurance payers.**

► **For fast payment, clean claims must be generated.**

► **Clean claims result from sound preregistration, insurance verification and coding processes.**

► **ECS will aid in identifying problem claims, while expediting cash and lowering cost.**

► **Insurance claim follow-up is necessary to release problem claims.**

► **The DOC approach to collections is a highly effective three-step process for collection follow-up staff.**

► **For payer system problems, work out the claims problem *en masse* with the payer's provider representative.**

To Do List

❑ Identify your top five reasons for payer rejections and prioritize the list by dollar impact.

❑ Resolve the top rejection reason.

❑ Find out from your practice management software vendor how they can help you implement an ECS process for your top five payers.

❑ Train your staff on the DOC approach to collections.

❑ Call in the provider representative of the payer with the highest percent of dollars over 90 days.

Answer These Questions About "Our Practice":

❑ Do you have a prebill editor (or editing system)?

❑ Do you have the name and phone number of your provider representative for all your major payers? When was the last time you talked with them?

❑ How do you know if your collection staff is effective?

Key Action Step 6
DEVELOP A HIGHLY EFFECTIVE AND EFFICIENT SELF-PAY COLLECTION PROGRAM

"*O*ur Practice" is having severe problems with its "self-pay" accounts. "Self-pay" refers to both the noninsured patients' liability and the patients' self-pay "portion" of the account not paid by their insurance(s). Exhibit 6.1 demonstrates the seriousness of the situation — on average, it is taking 272.3 days to collect the self-pay accounts.

Exhibit 6.1   Average days to collect self-pay accounts

	Net Accounts Receivable	Net Accounts Receivable Mix	Net Revenue	Net Revenue Mix	Day's Revenue	NDRO
Self-Pay	$1,425,000	30%	$157,000	10%	$5,233	272.3

By subjecting the self-pay financial class to our *Cash Opportunity* model, it would appear we have $666,161 in uncollected cash.

Each Day's Net Revenue (potential cash)	$5,233
Net Day's Revenue Outstanding — Current	272.3
Net Day's Revenue Outstanding — Goal	45.0
Net Day's Revenue Outstanding — Opportunity	127.3

Cash Opportunity = EAQ Day's Net Revenue* Net Day's Revenue Outstanding - Opportunity

Cash Opportunity	$666,161

Unfortunately, at this aging elevation, it is a sure thing many of these dollars are "dead" and uncollectible. Are you really going to bill someone for $35.00 on a bill that is three years old? Are they still at the same address? Maybe the patient's insurer really should have paid the claim. But what are the chances an insurance company will pay on any account over a year old? Or maybe some of the dollars are contractual allowances that were never written-off? Well, now you need to write them off. In any case, you have a problem.

Here's the problem

Self-pay is extremely troublesome for practices because they are "low dollar, high volume accounts." This mixture, unless tightly controlled, will, over time, clog your receivables. If you tried to have an intervention on each account, the small unit amount and the volumes involved would take a high investment in personnel, sinking your expense budget.

> *The best time for direct collection has come and gone. You had your best opportunity when the patient was standing in front of you. The next best opportunity for direct collect activity will be when the patient comes back for service. Direct collecting after service is costly and less effective than in person.*

A self-pay collection program which effectively and efficiently pursues "large" dollar balances needs to be implemented. The strategy will entail "sizing" the number of account dollars which are economically feasible to directly pursue and creating a high energy, well trained collection staff. The other tool of a self-pay collection strategy is the statement cycle, which will be discussed in Key Action Step 7.

A word of caution

It might seem like the same thing, but customer service calls (incoming) and patient follow-up calls (outgoing) differ from one another. Incoming calls prioritize the collector's time, outgoing calls are prioritized by the collector.

By mixing these two separate functions, the dollars pursued will not be prioritized. The patient calling in may want to discuss a $39.00 payment while a $1,200 account goes untouched. In the course of a day, staff trying to do both functions may — even if they are really good — make only 15 outgoing, prioritized calls a day compared with the 45 to a high of 100 needed to cost justify a follow-up collection staff.

Separate these functions. As long as these functions are combined, goals can not be developed because staff is unable to have full control over their time — or success.

Why are they calling? If your incoming call volumes are overwhelming, it is time to do an audit of the calls. Log in the reasons and the time it takes to resolve the patients' concerns. Typically, they are calling in because something is not working in your system.

Sizing the collection effort

There are two ways to approach the number of self-pay accounts you will pursue. The first is based on account dollar, that is, all accounts which exceed a certain dollar amount. The second approach is to determine the accounts pursued based on the staff available. The first approach assumes you will adjust your staffing to meet the volumes; the second approach assumes you will adjust your volumes to meet your staffing.

Approach number 1: Dollar amounts to be collected

At a certain dollar amount, it is not economically viable to pursue the account with collector activity. Whether this dollar value is $75 or $100 or $250 will depend on your patients' interest to pay, on your collectors' effectiveness and on the specialty of your practice. A $75 account may be economically viable only if your collector needs to make one phone call. With each no-contact call, each payment promise broken, the cost to collect rises above $75.

Analysis report:

> ▶ Exclude all accounts under $25.
> ▶ Report on accounts in aging category 30-90 days. This indicates accounts which are not being paid via statement processing.
> ▶ Identify total number of account balances.
> ▶ Identify total dollars.
> ▶ Identify average account balance.

With these volume numbers you have the data necessary to determine adequate staffing. Add our productivity standards to this analysis. The account contact productivity standard per-day per-collector is between a minimum of 45 to a high of 100. Contacts in this case include voice messages left. We also assume an average of 2.5 contacts per resolved account.

Exhibit 6.2 Volume numbers to determine adequate staffing

Self-pay Staff Resource Calculation (Excludes account under $25)		
Total dollars (agings 30-90 days) =		$58,480
Total accounts (agings 30-90 days) =		680
Average dollar per account (agings 30-90 days) = $58,480 / 780 =		**86**
Daily Productivity Target per one FTE per day		70
Average work days per month		20
Monthly Productivity Target per one FTE = 70 * 20 =		**1,400**
Average contacts per resolved account =		2.5
Total monthly contacts required = 2.5 * 680 (total accounts) =		1,700
Total FTE's necessary = $\dfrac{\text{Total monthly contacts required}}{\text{Monthly Productivity Target}}$ = $\dfrac{1700}{1400}$		**1.21**

As Exhibit 6.2 demonstrates, based on our volume statistics and productivity assumptions, we will need to attempt 1,700 contacts per month. One collector is able (based on a standard of 70 contacts per day) to accomplish 1,400 per month. Therefore, "Our Practice" will need to staff 1.21 collectors.

Approach number 2: Available staff

This approach entails that you will pursue as many accounts as there is staff. "Our Practice" will be able to staff only one-half FTE. From the previous analysis, you know that a collector should be able to make contact on 1,400 accounts per month. Therefore, a one-half FTE should be able to handle 700 accounts per month.

Go to your aged trial balance (ATB). Have it sorted from highest dollar account to lowest for self-pay accounts in aging bucket 30 to 90 days. Count down 700 accounts. Identify the dollar amount at the 700th selection. This is your approximate dollar limit.

Creating a high energy collections staff

Self-pay cash collection rests on hiring well, followed with training on effective collection techniques. When screening applicants for collector positions, it is important to look for certain traits. Top candidates are:

▶ Pleasant personalities who like working *with* people

▶ People with common and street sense who do not rely on strict rules but find solutions in the "real world"

▶ Competitive spirits who like to win within the rules

▶ People who present themselves well to the public—they have a bit of the actor in them

▶ Self-starters who will challenge you to keep up with them

▶ Prior collection experience in a medical practice environment

Developing good collectors

Collection is an art, not a science. It is the art of persuasion: giving the patient information to make informed decisions about how they will make payment. It is not learned quickly nor can it be practiced in a mechanical or indifferent way. As in insurance collection, the DOC approach is our framework for successful collections: 1) get to the decision maker, 2) overcome the obstacles and 3) gain a commitment.

To be efficient and effective, the collectors need to keep the following points taped to their desk:

▶ **Be brief.** Do not prolong a collection call with conversational chatter. Terminate the call as soon as possible while practicing good public relations techniques.

▶ **Do not argue.** You may win the argument but will lose the war—either through bad public relations or lost patient.

▶ **Use intelligence, not emotion.** An emotional collector is one who is no longer in control of the situation.

▶ **Sound (and be) confident.** This communicates authority and will command respect.

▶ **Be businesslike.** Organize the facts before the call is made.

▶ **Be friendly, but not familiar.** Firmness is more convincing when coupled with a formal tone.

▶ **Be courteous.** Always.

▶ **Be flexible.** You are dealing with human beings that have different needs and will be persuaded in different ways.

▶ **Be natural.** Use simple, uncomplicated sentences. Make your delivery unhurried and deliberate.

The call

Being unable to make contact with the patient is the greatest frustration of self-pay collections. To enhance the probability of contact, practices must arrange their hours of collection to coincide with when the patient is most likely be at home. With so many two-wage earner families, it is a requirement to concentrate collection activity in the evenings (M-Th) and Saturday mornings.

Every phone call should follow a standard format. Every call the collector should:

- ▶ Identify themselves by name and title
- ▶ Identify the organization
- ▶ State the reason for the call
- ▶ Indicate the bill is delinquent
- ▶ State the balance due
- ▶ Ask whether payment in full will be paid by cash, credit card or check
- ▶ Wait for a response. The patient's response will tell you what you need to know to collect the account.

Overcoming common obstacles — a few tips

The patient is aggressive. A request for payment may result in an unanticipated and unwarranted aggressive response from the patient. They may become abusive, calling the entire service received into question. Do not respond in kind! Express pleasure at hearing the complaints — listen intently to define the exact reason of their behavior. The situation may be resolved by a simple apology for a misunderstanding perceived or a discussion of options available to work out a financial problem may be in order.

Pleas for sympathy. Do not dispute the details of the story. Sympathy should be expressed, as well as a willingness to work out the financial arrangements of their bill. Make sure you reach an agreement with payment specifics.

Denial and evasion. Some patients will deny knowledge of a claim. Do not try to prove them wrong. Rather, restate the facts: date(s) of service, reason for the visit, physician's name and any other information the patient may desire. Then, request immediate payment.

Defiance. The patient may say, "So what?" and dare you to collect the bill. Now is the time to maintain your composure — keep in command of the situation. Make a direct request for payment. If the patient simply refuses to pay, state that if payment is not made within 10 days you will be given no option but to refer the account to a collection agency. Also, indicate if the patient wishes service in the future, they will need to pay all back balances plus a $50.00 prepayment. This is probably not the kind of patient you want.

Interviewing techniques

The ability to interview patients about their bill is essential to successful collections. Sound interviewing techniques will help determine the facts and set the stage for working with the patient toward account resolution.

Interviewing also allows the collector to be in control of the collection call. As the interviewer, a leadership role is established and the conversation can be guided to productive areas.

In the interview, use questions with "who," "what," "when," "where" and "why." These types of questions require more than a "yes" or "no" answer and may reveal why the patient is not paying. Questions find out what will motivate payment.

Choice-option questions

"Choice-option" questions allow the patient to select between alternatives. It provides them the respect of not being told what to do. Patients can be asked:

▶ "Yes, I understand your situation. Would you like to make the final payment in 10 days or would the end of the month be more convenient?" (This conversation assumes "...the end of the month..." is what you would like as the outcome.)

▶ "Do you want to pay by cash, check or credit card?"

▶ "Would it be more convenient for you to drop the payment in the mail today, or would you like to stop by the office this afternoon?"

Giving patients the choice yields great results, just make sure the worse case option is advantageous to the practice.

Just say no to "no"

"No" is a forbidden word. Your staff must use caution so questions do not result in the patient saying "no" to paying. When a patient is asked, "Will you be sending payment today?" it is too easy for the patient to say "no." Try, "When will you be sending payment?"

Using questions and allowing patients to tell their story and come to their own decisions is the most effective collection tool available. Questions break the *indifference barrier*. Once a patient's indifference to making payment is broken through, payment is not far behind.

Exhibit 6.3 Motivator topics for collecting

Topic	Leads patient to...
Good credit rating	...understand good credit rating is a valuable asset. This conversation will usually occur as the patient realizes if payment is not forthcoming, they will be going off to a collection agency.
Responsibility	...understand how the physician was there for them when their health was in question. The physician has expended resources on their behalf and it is only fair — and cost effective — to keep up their end of the relationship.
Freedom from worry	...an awareness of payment options. Emphasized options are provided as a courtesy because the practice does not want patients worrying about their financial commitments.
Appreciation	...appreciate the unique relationship of the patient and physician. Explain the physician values the relationship and it is only fair to appreciate the physician's commitment. (As last resort, explain to patient if they are unable to reciprocate and support the physician, then maybe the relationship is not a good one).
Added costs	...be aware of late charges if payment is not received. (In your payment authorization, there should be language authorizing the charging of interest and late charges.)

Goal setting

As in insurance follow-up, goals need to be set, monitored and rewarded — both individually and as a group. Establish a goal for each collector to make contact with at least 70 patients a day with at least 35 resolved per eight-hour period. Identify the largest dollar balances and set a cash dollar amount to accompany the number of resolved accounts. Project this amount out for a monthly collector goal and summarize it for a total group goal.

Have each collector fill out a Collection Action Report daily. (See page 43 as part of Key Action Step 5.) This report is crucial in establishing that the collector resolved the account — that is, reached an agreement with the patient — which will ultimately result in payment. This report establishes that goals are being met and ensures the staff understands the DOC approach to account resolution.

Review the reports in short, weekly meetings. Discussing specific problems and collection effectiveness techniques should become an agenda item of these staff meetings. Make sure when goals are reached, they are appropriately celebrated and incentives are distributed.

Exhibit 6.4   Goals to implement — self-pay collections

> ❏ **Individual**
>
> > ❏ Highest dollar volume collected
> >
> > ❏ Greatest percentage increase in dollars collected (to motivate improved performance)
> >
> > ❏ Highest volume collected each day or weekly (to maintain ongoing enthusiasm)
>
> ❏ **Team**
>
> > ❏ Monthly cash goal
> >
> > ❏ Reduction in bad debt expense—Year-to-date
> >
> > ❏ Dollars over 90 days under 10 percent (Not including installment plans)
> >
> > ❏ Reduction in dollars over 90 days (to motivate improved team performance)

Goal setting will not only increase collections but establishes a framework for success. Staff will understand and appreciate what success is and how to achieve it. When they meet the goals, they will have an objective basis from which *they know* they are respected for their competencies. A combination of team and individual incentives will promote team spirit while individual excellence is recognized. This discussion will be expanded in the Key Action Step 12 titled "The Implementation Plan And Motivation For Results."

Collection effectiveness

As with your insurance collection staff, a *Payment History Analysis* needs to be undertaken on a regular basis. Select ten accounts at random for each member of the collection staff. Review each account to determine:

> ➤ When the collection follow-up started
>
> ➤ If collector made contact with decision maker; if not, did collector use sound judgement on keeping account on active Accounts Receivable (i.e., not writing it off to collection agency)
>
> ➤ If collector overcame the obstacles
>
> ➤ If full payment or partial payment is received for self-pay accounts (Are small monthly payments accepted too easily?)
>
> ➤ Is collector able to make decision on account status or is collector prone to accepting delays without subsequent payment? (Constant callbacks and lack of reason for delays should be noted. Is the collector trying to settle too quickly or accepting the easy way out too often?)

- ▶ If there are too many "no contact" or "left message" (This would probably indicate the hours of collection are ineffective. Try nights and Saturday morning.)
- ▶ If there is *too much follow-up activity* on a consistent basis (This is a sign the contact is not effective. The collector probably needs additional training in closing the account.)
- ▶ If payment promises are monitored (Calls need to be made on the date, or day after, of the promise.)
- ▶ If collector is getting agreement on payment or an alternative course of action
- ▶ A specific date
- ▶ If a specific, clear and understandable agreement was reached
- ▶ If collector memoed system effectively and efficiently

The reviews need to be shared with the individual collector. Common problems shared by the collection staff should be quantified and discussed at team meetings.

A helpful training tool is monitoring collection calls. This will lead to immediate feedback through collegial discussion. Use the same key points noted above for the discussion points.

The Fair Debt Collection Practices Act

The Fair Debt Collection Practices Act, which became law on March 20, 1978, was designed to stop abusive collection practices by third party, professional debt collectors. Legally the Act is not binding on "...any officer or employee of a creditor while, in the name of the creditor, collecting debts for such collector." (FDCPA—Section 803.6(A)) However, abusive practices are not in the best interest of anyone and the provisions of the Act give a solid guideline for effective and fair collection practices.

Requirements of the act you should be aware of

If mailings are used to verify a debtor's location, any language or symbol indicating that the communication relates to the collection of a debt should be omitted from the stationery and envelope. The law also prohibits using a postcard to correct location information. In locating a debtor, the collector is prohibited by law from communicating with a third party more than once, unless expressly requested to do so by that party, or the collector believes the first response was erroneous or incomplete.

Once the collector knows the consumer is represented by an attorney with respect to the debt and knows the name and address of that attorney, the collector must not communicate with anyone else, "unless the attorney fails to respond within a reasonable period of time." The law does not provide specific parameters for a " reasonable period of time." For protection of a medical group in lawsuits, it is good to establish a written office policy which can be used as a defense.

Within five days after the initial communication, the collector is obligated to send the debtor written verification of the amount of the debt and the creditor to whom the debt is owed. If the debtor makes a written request for information or disputes any portion of the debt within 30 days, the collector must cease collection of the debt, or any disputed portion thereof. The Fair Credit Billing Act, a part of the Consumer Credit Protection Act of 1968, defines guidelines similar to those specified in this section of the Fair Debt Collection Practices Act (American Collector's Association, Inc., 1979).

The law places limitations on communication with the debtor. Generally, the debt collector may only contact a patient between 8 A.M. and 9 P.M. in the debtor's time zone, unless the collector is aware that the patient works at night and sleeps during the day, or is otherwise inconvenienced by receiving communications during that time period. Collectors may not call patients at work if they know or have reason to know the debtor's employer prohibits such communications.

Once a consumer notifies the collector in writing not to contact them, the collector must cease all communications. However, the collector may make one last communication but only to advise collection efforts are being terminated and/or to make notification legal remedies may or will be invoked.

"A debt collector may not engage in any conduct for which the natural consequence is to harass, oppress or abuse any person in connection with the collection of a debt," says the law (Ibid.). Six specific instances of abuse are expressly prohibited, but they are not all-inclusive. These are:

▶ Use or threat of violence or other criminal means to harm the physical person, reputation or property.
▶ Use of obscene, profane or abusive language.
▶ Publication of "debtor lists." (Names of consumers who do not pay can be distributed to consumer reporting agencies.)
▶ Advertisement of the sale of any debt to coerce payment of the debt.
▶ Causing a telephone to ring or engaging any person in telephone conversation repeatedly or continuously with intent to annoy, abuse or harass.
▶ Placement of telephone calls without meaningful disclosure of the caller's identity.

The law prohibits any false representation intended to mislead the debtor, such as distorting company documents in such a way as to make the reader believe they are legal documents, falsifying the collector's identity, misstating the nature or status of a debt or any other misleading designations.

The law specifically prohibits some unfair practices. Included are such practices as: depositing a postdated check prior to the date on the check; causing collect charges on a telephone bill, telegram expenses, or other costs to be made to the consumer; or, using a post card to communicate with a consumer.

The Fair Debt Collection Practices Act is enforced both administratively and judicially. The Federal Trade Commission can treat a violation of the act as an unfair or deceptive practice under the law. Violators are also subject to civil penalties in federal and state courts.

SUMMARY OF KEY ACTION STEP 6

➤ Self-pay collection is problematic because they are often low dollar, high volume. A collection strategy which is aware of the cost to collect is necessary.

➤ The most effective and least costly time for direct collections is at the time of service.

➤ It is important to "size" your self-pay collection effort.

➤ A well-trained collection staff using the DOC approach will result in increased cash while enhancing customer satisfaction.

➤ Goals are critical to success. Setting and monitoring goals will lead to increased cash collections.

➤ By tracking collectors' performances, it will allow for incentives to be awarded, system obstacles identified and, if necessary, additional training to take place.

➤ Training collectors on collection techniques consistent with favorable public relations is essential to successful management of a practice.

➤ It should always be kept in mind that the job of collectors is to collect, sell and motivate—not downgrade and humiliate.

➤ Incorporating effective questioning techniques into the collection approach will produce positive results.

To Do List

❑ Estimate size of self-pay follow-up effort and necessary staffing levels

❑ Audit of accounts of self-pay collectors for DOC method

❑ Schedule staff for evening and Saturday morning collection efforts

❑ Meet with staff for goal setting

Questions To Ask About "Our Practice":

❑ How many payment resolutions are your collectors accomplishing a day?

❑ What is the lowest dollar balance the collectors pursue?

❑ Do you fit the size of the collection task to staff or the size of staff to the collection task?

❑ What is your average self-pay balance?

❑ Why weren't these dollars collected at time of service?

Key Action Step 7
TIGHTEN STATEMENT CYCLE TO ENHANCE PATIENT CASH AT LOW COST

The problem with collecting self-pay balances — as discussed in Key Action Step 6 — is trying to manage high-volume, small-balance accounts in a cost effective manner. It is not feasible to intervene on every account. In fact, it is not feasible to have staff intervene on 80 percent of accounts. The cost of trying to collect a $10 account is identical to a $150 account. You will lose money on every $10 account you try to collect.

The only way to make feasible the collection of small-balance, self-pay accounts is to design a statement processing cycle which is both effective and efficient. In chapter 6 we have already "sized" the accounts "Our Practices" collection staff is able to handle. The rest will be handled through statement notifications.

The theory behind statements

A statement is a communication. It informs the patient that a specific dollar amount is required by a specific date. The first communication sent is a reminder for payment. Most patients, because they are used to getting bills and paying, will pay immediately off this first statement.

After the first statement, the game changes. If there is no payment within 15 days from receipt, alarms should go off. Because most people pay on the first notice, nonpayment means the patient has to be motivated to make payment. Each communication after the first needs to increase the sense of urgency.

The second statement communications must tell the patient the account is delinquent and seriously past due. Unless payment is received within 15 days, there will be consequences.

What happens if no payment is received after the second communication? First of all, it is now confirmed this account is a collection problem. Second, unless the sense of urgency is radically heightened, sending out statements three, four or five will be useless.

It is recommended, after the second statement, a "precollect" letter is sent. A precollect is a letter sent from a third party (i.e., many collection agencies offer this service and there are dedicated precollect companies) which indicates the account has been referred to the precollect service for collection. Although the account is still on your active accounts receivable, the patient realizes their unpaid account is being special handled because it is delinquent and the sense of urgency has been taken to a new level.

Precollect letters can be one letter, two letters or more. It is recommended that at least two be used. The first precollect would indicate the account has been referred and that it is serious. The second or final would be to inform the patient the account is being sent to collections. It also states the account will be referred in 10 days unless the patient intervenes.

The referral to a collection agency is the highest elevation of urgency you are able to invoke. In Key Action Step 9, we will discuss the effective use of collection agencies.

Exhibit 7.1 provides recommended statement cycles activities and timing. It is recommended to add a "dummy" account in your name to the practice management system to verify timely processing. Exhibits 7.2 and 7.3 offers some possibilities on statement wording.

Exhibit 7.1   Possible statement cycle

Days from initial statement	Billing cycle item
	Initial statement
30 days	2nd statement
45 days	1st precollect
60 days	2nd precollect
75 days	Refer to agency

Exhibit 7.2   Sample statement messages

Message #1	Please mail in full payment today.
Message #2	This balance is past due. Please pay promptly and avoid further action.
Message #3	This balance is seriously past due. Unless you pay immediately, we will be referring your account for special handling in 10 days.

Exhibit 7.3 Sample messages — no response from insurance

Message #1	No insurance payment received. Please call your insurance company.
Message #2	Your insurance has not paid bill. We now consider this bill to be your responsibility. Please pay immediately.
Message #3	This balance is seriously past due. Unless you pay immediately, we will be referring your account for special handling in 10 days.

The "information-only statement" — Yes or No?

Should the practice send information to patients when no payment is requested (i.e., "Our Practice has billed your insurance company—no payment is required at this time") or should it send statements only when a payment is requested?

There are two kinds of people in this world—those who send statements only when an action is required by the patient and those who will send statements to keep the patient informed on the status of their account. It is costly to send statements on an "information only" basis and many times it only confuses the patient ("Am I supposed to do something with this statement?"). However, many practices believe keeping the patient fully informed is part of their customer service mission. Because of the cost and because it does not enhance cash flow, it is not recommended.

Statements that work

Because of the large-volume, low-dollar accounts, statements must be as effective as possible. Patients often complain that health care statements are difficult to understand, confusing or do not provide enough information. The following tips will help in the design of effective "patient friendly" notices or statements which will support "Our Practice's" public relation goals:

➤ Keep statements simple. Avoid unnecessary words or information that will confuse the reader.

➤ Include all pertinent information regarding the account (date of service, balance, account number) without overloading the notice with data.

➤ Include a return envelope to make it easy for the patient to send payment.

➤ Be direct, but avoid any confrontational language.

➤ Be sure the statement clearly points out that the medical group accepts credit cards as a payment option. If possible, include a tear-off section for the patient to write in credit card information.

➤ Notices should be geared toward obtaining payment in full rather than payment arrangements.

➤ The messages on notices should clearly state the status of the patient's account.

The desired action required of the patient is communicated through both word and the graphic design of the statement itself. The following design elements will emphasize your message:

➤ **Size** — Use larger fonts to increase attention to important information elements and to recognize the aging of a patient population.

➤ **Motion** — Use motion through the use of arrows, ellipses or other symbols to draw the eye towards the important elements of the notice.

- ▶ **Isolation** — Important information or instructions need to stand in isolation to command attention. Notice design needs to be free of clutter.

- ▶ **Color** — The eye is drawn towards the red end of the color spectrum. Oranges, reds, yellows and pinks should be utilized for important information elements.

SUMMARY OF KEY ACTION STEP 7

➤ Rely on statement processing for all high-volume, low-dollar accounts.

➤ A tight statement cycle will expedite cash.

➤ Most people who plan on paying will pay from first statement.

➤ If form letters will be used in follow-up, design them with care, keeping both collection and public relations in mind.

➤ Keep form letters and statements simple.

To Do List

❑ Review current statement cycle

❑ Investigate how to change statement messages, number of accounts and spacing between accounts

❑ Model the statement cycle which maximizes cash flow and minimizes cost while maintaining or enhancing customer service to reproduce

❑ Add a dummy name mailed to yourself to verify timely processing.

Answer These Questions About "Our Practice":

❑ When was the last time you reviewed your statement messages?

❑ When was the last time you modified your statement cycle?

❑ Based on patient comments, are your statements confusing?

Key Action Step 8
A MANAGED CARE STRATEGY

"Our Practice" has 12 percent of its net revenue under managed care contracts. Managed care, from an accounts receivable standpoint, is a reimbursement model that imposes upon the provider responsibilities for utilization management (UM). The economic rationale for managed care is health care costs can be controlled through a reduction in services while maintaining the quality of care.

The utilization requirements are the heart of managed care. In the classic managed care model, the primary care physician is the "gatekeeper," and decides if referrals to a specialist are necessary. To document approval has been given for additional services, a referral is created with copies to the specialist and to the HMO utilization review (UR) staff.

If significant services involving high cost procedures or services are involved, the managed care contract may detail that pre-authorizations are necessary before the procedure can be performed. Additionally, inpatient hospital services often involve a "concurrent review" before approval of additional days is granted.

The basic model is rather simple but, because of the UM requirements, there is a high risk of denials and payment delays. "Our Practice" is struggling to fulfill the UM requirements and has been forced to "write-off" dollars denied due to non-compliance. To be successful,"Our Practice" must address the following areas:

▶ The contract
▶ Living the contract
▶ Monitoring managed care payments and denials
▶ Patient education

The contract

Too often managed care contracts are signed without any input from the people who will have to administer the partnership. It should be a requirement that all contracts are at least reviewed and discussed among practice staff so potential problems are identified for the contract negotiators. However, formal review by an expert with experience in managed care contract analysis is strongly recommended.

When reviewing the contract, here is a list of items you will want to ensure are included (or excluded) in the contract.

▶ Thoroughly review the utilization review requirements. Do they place an unreasonable burden on your operations?

▶ Is there language which allows the payer to deny claims for individual lapses?

▶ Remove language which allows unilateral denial of claims for individual lapses. Build in language which mandates there must be "…ongoing, persistent nonconformance behaviors which are economically damaging…" before the managed care company is allowed to deny claim payments.

▶ Make sure there is a clause which mandates there will be no retroactive denials for authorizations granted.

▶ Build in language which allows pre-authorization requests to be faxed to the managed care firm with returned approvals within two hours.

▶ Make sure you are able to resolve payment problems with the patient. Include the clause, "…Contact with the patient will be allowed … when payment or a written denial have not been received within the payment term."

▶ In the Dispute Resolution section, allow for the ability to resolve the entire class of delinquent claims. Also, include language indicating defining the mechanism for advanced funding for payer system failures or delinquencies.

▶ Contractually obligate the payer to have subscriber cards current and distributed to subscribers.

▶ Define all services where attachments to the HCFA 1500 are required.

▶ For claim resolution, require that an individual with authority to approve claim payments be dedicated to "Our Practice's" account.

▶ Require payer to provide in service for staff on billing requirements.

▶ Require standing receivables meetings designed to resolve delinquent claims and system issues.

Make sure you become a player in designing the operational contract. The negotiator needs to be aware of problems being experienced with existing contracts. Include an analysis of the amount of dollars being denied and withheld due to contractual problems. More information on managed care contracting can be found in the recently published MGMA Center for Research handbook titled *Financial Management for Medical Groups*. See the referral to titles in the back of this book.

Living the contract

It is critical the contract in its entirety be explained to the people who need to administer its financial terms. This will be critical in ensuring that the UM documentation is in place, demanding that payment requirements are adhered to and accurately discussing the contract obligations with the patient.

Managed care UM requirements emphasize the importance of pregistration and insurance verification. This is to address and resolve any problems with respect to the patient being "out of network" (i.e., they are trying to see a physician who is not under contract with their managed care company), referrals not being in place and pre-authorization for service not being approved.

If they are not resolved prior to service, patient complaints will mount and payment denials will increase. Exhibit 8.1 lists common reasons for managed care denials that are related to poor execution of contract terms.

Everyone of these reasons for "denial" is alleviated by a sound "front-end" with strong preregistration and insurance verification protocols.

Exhibit 8.1 Common reasons for managed care denial

Denial reason	Possible explanantion
Sent to wrong carrier	Incorrect insurance plan code
Provider is not a member of the managed care network	Staff is not familiar with health care organization's managed care contract or provider is not appropriately credentialed
Patient not eligible at time of service	Staff did not call to verify eligibility of the patient prior to service
Authorization not obtained prior to service	Staff either not familiar with which procedures require authorization or did not obtain the authorization
Unable to identify subscriber	Staff may not have entered the correct social security number, policy number or employer name of the subscriber
Failure to notify payer of patient's admission within specified time frame	Staff did not call the managed care organization within the specified time frame
Service not covered	Staff did not obtain benefit information and patient received services not covered by his/her payer

Monitoring managed care payments

From both a cash flow and financial control standpoint, monitoring of managed care contracts is required. The complexities of some managed care contracts, coupled with limitations in both payer and provider systems, make the probability of incorrect payments extremely high.

The most effective and efficient method of ensuring correct payments is through the use of your system's "contractual reimbursement master" — if your practice management software has this capability. This profile contains the reimbursement terms of each of your contracts. At the time of billing, the system writes off any contractual allowances stating the receivable as the expected payment. At the time of payment, the cash application staff will be able to see if the payment matches the receivable.

The problem with the automated system approach is the amount of effort it takes to set up the system. A person knowledgeable in system profiles, as well as contract terms, must take charge of this process and be dedicated to its success. However, while the first time is the hardest, the effort will pay off in staff productivity and payment accuracy.

If your system is unable to accommodate your contracts, a manual review of payment accuracy is required. In this scenario, the cash application staff must be thoroughly versed in the reimbursement terms of the contract.

Reimbursement methodologies

There are four major reimbursement methodologies:

Fee schedules — The payer is charged according to a fee schedule set for each service and/or procedure to be provided. This fee-for-service arrangement is low risk.

Percentage discount — A discount on charges. From the practice's standpoint, this is a low risk contract as long as the discounted fee still covers the entire cost of service. This is a fee-for-service arrangement.

Global fee — This structure is used in higher-intensity services, such as surgical procedures. It pays a fixed priced based on an International Classification of Diseases, Ninth Revision (ICD-9) procedure code, regardless of the amount of supplies given or time spent. This type of contract is high risk for the provider since any time or service over a "norm" will be at the expense of the practice.

Capitation — Under a capitated arrangement, a monthly capitated rate ("per-member per-month" or PMPM) is paid to a physician based on the number of members which designated that physician as their primary care physician. The capitated payment covers all services for all the members' services. This is the highest risk arrangement to the practice. "Our Practice" needs to carefully assess if it has all systems in place to successfully engage in capitation. Effective management of capitation contracts requires highly sophisticated financial management systems and experienced staff to control associated risks.

Patient education and managed care

Because of the responsibilities placed on the provider and the patient for UM, patient education is critical in reducing financial risk. Patient and physician (and the physician's staff) must understand the contract they signed. The areas that need to be addressed are:

► Utilization management

► Access to physicians, services and facilities

► In-network and out-of-network fees

► Pre-authorization requirements

► Financial liability, including a patient's co-payment, deductible and patient's portion for noncovered services.

It does not matter that it may be the patient's responsibility to know the terms of their insurance benefits. The patient's perspective is that the physician and office staff should know their (the patient's) coverage and responsibilities. Even though the patient may be responsible the practice will share in lost reimbursement due to denials for noncompliance.

In situations where services are not available to the patient because of UM guidelines, there will be situations where the patient will need counseling. Listed below are ways to assist the patient with potential denials.

► **Explain alternatives.** Inform patients that a denial does not prohibit them from receiving treatment. In a specialist's office, the patient may only need to receive a referral from their primary physician. The patient may also opt to proceed with treatment, with the understanding they will be responsible for the bill.

► **Offer member services to the patient.** In situations where the patient demands service, your only alternative is to get the patient talking with a representative from their managed care company

► **Field questions.** Always ask patients if there are any issues that you can clarify or answer. This is an opportunity to enhance patient satisfaction as well as helping the patient and staff to better understand confusing issues.

Selection of managed care organization types

HMO — A medical delivery system distributed through selected physicians and providers with a mission to provide quality healthcare through appropriate utilization controls. The primary care physician is the utilization "gatekeeper" with risk shifted to the physicians to encourage compliance.

Staff Model HMO — Type of HMO where utilization is controlled by employed physicians.

Group Model HMO — Type of HMO where the network is comprised of large multispecialty groups or clinics.

Independent Practice Association (IPA) — An association of independent physicians who negotiate contracts with HMOs as a group. Each physician retains his or her own practice. They are subject to the contracts the IPA signs.

Preferred Provider Organization (PPO) — Not an insurance company. A PPO is a negotiating and claim repricing entity which offers to self-insured employers or insurers a network of physicians and other providers at reduced rates. The insurance companies or third-party administrators (a company which processes claims and payments for a set fee) will distribute patient identification cards, process claims, and make payments.

Point-of-Service (POS) — Allows subscribers some coverage if they choose out-of-network providers. Going outside, however, will be at an increased out-of-pocket expense to the subscriber through increased deductibles and coinsurance. This type of HMO responds to the consumers' demand to have access to the physicians of their choice while allowing the higher cost to the consumer to act as a utilization control.

More information on types of managed care organizations are listed in the previously referenced *Financial Management for Medical Groups.*

SUMMARY OF KEY ACTION STEP 8

➤ Because of the contractual utilization requirements, managed care puts the practice at risk.

➤ All staff needs to be knowledgeable about contract terms to reduce the risk of denials and bill rejections.

➤ Patient education about the patient's obligations under their managed care contract is critical in reducing the risk under managed care contracts.

➤ Because of the high rate of inappropriately paid claims under managed care contracts, it is critical reimbursement is monitored at the time of cash posting.

➤ All contracts should be reviewed focusing on the ability to effectively administer the contract within the practice's operating procedures.

To Do List

❑ Gather all managed care contracts and create a working matrix detailing utilization review guidelines, referral processing, payment terms and payer contacts.

❑ Conduct training session with staff on the matrix.

❑ Identify all claims rejected for lack of pre-authorization or other utilization guidelines over the last six months.

❑ Talk to person who negotiates contracts and discuss with them importance of having insight from operations.

Answer These Questions About "Our Practice":

❑ Is your and physicians staff given the details about the managed care contracts to administer the contracts and provide quality patient education?

❑ When was the last time a managed care provider representative came to your site to do staff and physician education?

Key Action Step 9
MAXIMIZE COLLECTION AGENCY RECOVERY

As noted in "Our Practice's" *Aged Trial Balance* in Key Action Step 1, page 5, there is a huge problem with self-pay accounts not being worked. Potential for turning these accounts into cash without the assistance of a collection agency is small to none.

The use of collection agencies is an important component in a self-pay collection program. This key strategy will explain how to get the most out of external collection agencies. The choice of an agency and its performance will make a difference in cash flow and receivables efficiency.

When to refer an account to an outside agency

Decisive action is necessary when deciding when an account needs to be removed from active A/R and placed with an agency. Referring an account involves a cost ("contingency fee" of the account value), but there is also a cost associated with holding onto accounts when internal resources are not sufficient to extract payment.

There are three major points to consider when analyzing accounts receivables before referring them to an agency for collection. These are:

1. Economic factor

2. Time factor

3. Public relations factor

Economic factors

Three important economic questions should be asked before submitting any account to a collection agency:

► Are the agency's fees reasonable when contrasted with internal collection costs?

► Is invoking the heightened urgency of placement necessary for payment?

► Are internal resources sufficient to bring the requisite focus on this particular account?

Because of the high-volume, low-dollar value in most practices, it is not possible to directly intervene on the majority of accounts. At a certain dollar value it would cost more to collect the account than the value of the account. From an economic viewpoint, when internal collection costs make net recovery less than what is expected from an agency, it is time to refer the account to outside professional collectors.

Time factors

Staff resources are limited and there are accounts which, despite your best intentions, will never be pursued. There needs to be a date in which you will refer accounts aged over a certain number of days from the initial statement. Firm decisions must be made. In some cases, this might be 90 days or 120 days. In any case, an account should never age over 120 days before being turned over to an agency unless there are unusual factors that are approved by the practice administrator.

There is a time value of an account. The older it is, the greater probability it is uncollectible. Patients may move, become unemployed, or take on excessive debt. The key is to keep collection efforts consistent and timely.

Patient relations factors

Patient relations are a consideration. Referring an account to an agency is certainly not an honor. However, if you have notified the patient multiple times and there is no record of cooperation, the patient is at fault and is hurting the practice. Patients must act in accordance with your mission and procedures. Ask yourself: "Is it reasonable to expect patients to pay? Do we have financial options? Are we reasonable in our practices?"

The use of a collection agency will demonstrate to the patient sound business practices. To not pursue the account will, paradoxically, engender disrespect for shoddy practices — and encourage nonpaying patients to…not pay. You owe it to your other patients to implement tight but fair collection practices.

How to select an agency

Every practice must find an agency that it trusts. The collection agency is the agent of the practice and does its work in the name of the practice. The agent you choose must be ethical in its dealing with the patient and in its dealings with the practice. The best reference of long-term ethical dealings is the good word from its established clients, particularly medical group practices and other health care providers.

The Appendix contains "Collection Procedures and Practices for Collection Agencies." This provides a working document that can be used as a Request for Proposal for services from an agency.

It is recommended, unless you are a very large practice, to use only one agency. Even with only one agency, the dollars involved probably are not going to make you one of their larger clients. Splitting up your business will decrease your contribution to their bottom line and can make you a client of "lesser importance." Use what clout you have.

Commissions and recovery rate

Commissions

Agencies work on a contingent fee basis. If there is no collection, there is no charge. You may want to structure rates based on benchmarks, negotiate penalties for not meeting agreed recovery rates, and build in rewards for exceeding expectations.

Agencies will usually entertain the idea of reduced rates for early placements. The "younger" the account when placed, the lower the fee. Collection agencies understand the time value of accounts.

Payments collected by the practice need to be promptly communicated to the agency. Payments not communicated may result in further collection efforts and horrible public relations. "Our Practice" should set up an automated communications system.

Contingent fee commissions charged by agencies will depend on the average dollar amount placed and the age of the account when placed. Accounts requiring legal action, or accounts transferred to out-of-town agencies will command a higher percentage. Try to negotiate the best rate, but the most important is an effective rate of recovery.

The rate of recovery

The real test of an agency is not the commission but the rate of recovery. A low commission coupled with a low recovery rate is not the equation for success. The practice must find an agency that will supply the necessary resources to make collections while protecting its public image. The agency needs to make a fair profit to be successful. It may be advantageous to go with the agency charging the higher rate. The importance of the rate of recovery is illustrated by the agency comparison in Figure 9.1.

Exhibit 9.1   Comparison of collection agencies A and B

	Agency A	Agency B
Total dollars submitted	$25,000	$25,000
Gross amount collected	$15,000	$7,000
Percent recovery rate (collections to submissions)	60%	28%
Commissions paid	$5,250	$1,750
Percent paid (commissions to collections)	35%	25%
Total net recovery	$9,750	$5,250
Percent net recovery rate *	39%	21%

* Divide total net recovery by total dollars submitted.

Obviously, collection agency "A," while charging higher commissions, has a higher recovery rate which pays dividends to "Our Practice." The net recovery after commission is the key financial factor.

Regular listings and cancellation of accounts

Accounts should be listed on a regular basis with your agency. It is recommended groups transfer accounts to agencies at least weekly.

You have the right to cancel any account that has been placed with an agency. There may be instances of placing an account which, for public relations, you need to "close and return." You have the right and authority to cancel; they have the duty to please the customer — you.

The audit

The audit of your agency will confirm the agency's collection practices are consistent with the message "Our Practice" wants to portray to patients. The following tips offer advice on how to handle and what to look for in an agency audit:

▶ Bring a list of accounts to be audited.   Do not let the agency "prepare" the accounts. The list should include a mixture of paid accounts, accounts "closed and returned" as uncollectible, active accounts, and accounts approved for legal action.

▶ Review all dunning (statement) notices and the agency's collection policies to ensure they are consistent with the mission of "Our Practice."

▶ Note when the agency begins collection activity after placement.   An initial notice should be sent to the patient within one working day after the account is listed, and and followed up by a telephone contact within one week.

▶ If the patient has not been contacted, review the time of day when contact is attempted and the length of time between attempts.

▶ Review all collection activity on accounts which were "closed and returned" as uncollectible. Was the patient given enough opportunity to pay? Did the agency complete adequate "skip-tracing" (trying to locate the patient) steps?

▶ Look closely at the dollar amounts where only a collection letter was sent. An agency can only pursue dollar amounts with direct collector intervention at a certain minimum dollar — $50? $75? $100? Does this coincide with the dollar amount to which the agency has agreed?

▶ Review the paid accounts to the type of activity it is taking to receive payment. If the agency is experiencing a high return for rebilling third-party carriers to receive payment, it is wise to improve your own practice's billing and collection areas.

▶ On legal accounts, make certain the patient had sufficient opportunity to pay voluntarily. Legal action is costly and reduces the practice's net recovery. Thus have the agency take legal action only if absolutely necessary.

▶ Listen to collectors as they work your practice's accounts.

▶ Review with the collection supervisor and collector(s) any patient complaints received about their collection practices.

▶ Watch for small monthly payment plans without supporting financial documentation. All efforts for payment in full should be exhausted (credit card, bank financing, etc.). If a payment plan exceeds a certain time period (typically six months), be sure the agency has received your approval. If a small monthly payment plan is in place, the agency should also be encouraging the patient every few months to see if the debtor's financial situation has changed.

Although the collection agency is a separate organization, patients still view it as an extension of the medical group. While its tactics may be more aggressive than those of the medical group, the agency's actions must work under your guidelines for working with your patients.

Further considerations for working with your collection agency(s):

▶ Do not hesitate to have a particular collector removed if numerous complaints are received. Do not accept excuses why their actions were necessary.

▶ Your staff should not be spending excessive time copying or researching information on agency accounts. If this is the case, have someone from the agency on-site to do the research and copying.

> ► A maximum time limit (six months) can be set for collection efforts. This gives the agency an incentive to collect quickly.

Attorneys for collection

Who gets better collection results — collection agencies or attorneys? If volume is the only criteria, the answer is collection agencies. However, some medical groups are using attorneys for collection services. Assuming contingency fees for collection activity are competitively priced, there are some definite benefits to this approach:

> ► Impact on patients when a letter is received from an attorney
> ► Patient perspective that this matter is more serious
> ► Attorney's ability to file suit quicker and for less cost
> ► Attorney's ability to spread legal costs over numerous accounts
> ► Ability of attorney to deal with other attorneys in accident cases

Most collection agencies will offer legal services. The collection agent who provides the best net return is the one to use.

Importance of analysis

It is important to do a yearly analysis of your agency. If the rate of return is less than expected, it may be time to investigate another agency. However, it is important you have discussed goals and expectations with your agency. They will have ideas as to how to improve their rate of collection.

SUMMARY OF KEY ACTION STEP 9

▶ A collection agency is a representative (an "agent") of the practice.

▶ A collection agency is useful in heightening the urgency of a delinquent account.

▶ Policies and procedures need to be developed to ensure accounts are referred on a timely basis.

▶ An outside agency should be chosen carefully. The agency should not only be able to demonstrate excellent collection rates and competitive commissions, but it must also have a reputation for being ethical.

▶ Any agency should demonstrate a patient relations policy compatible with your own practice's philosophy.

▶ Goal setting is required to obtain desired results.

▶ Monitoring and auditing collection agency activities is required in obtaining better results.

▶ Periodic evaluations should be part of the agreement with the agency.

To Do List

❑ Invite your current agency to develop goals based on the practice's cash needs, the quality of the accounts being referred and the techniques employed by the agency.

❑ Conduct an audit of your agency(s).

❑ Calculate the net recovery rate of your agency(s).

Answer These Questions About "Our Practice":

❑ Do you trust your agency(s)?

❑ Are you more concerned about the commission rate or the recovery rate?

❑ On average, at what day do you turn your accounts over to your agency? From the agency's point of view, is this too early? Too late?

Key Action Step 10
TAKE ADVANTAGE OF THE ELECTRONIC WORLD FOR PRODUCTIVITY, ACCURACY AND CASH ACCELERATION

An operational review of "Our Practice" reveals that use of its practice management system and technology available to increase cash flow, raise the productivity of staff and aid in accuracy of data is minimal at best. Caught in the past, "Our Practice" is struggling to keep up with increased volumes — and word has it that two new physicians will be added within six months. What then?

Envision this world

► After a patient is registered, a subscriber's eligibility and benefit level is verified electronically.

► Your system automatically, at the time of billing, posts any contractual discounts and sets the account to the expected payment.

► The claim, after it passes an internal prebill edit, is electronically submitted to the payer.

► The payer, after its internal edits, creates an online edit file which is used by your staff to correct.

► The payer submits an electronic remittance (EOB) file which is posted to your system.

► Statements are submitted via a file to an "electronic print shop" which prints, folds, stuffs and mails the statements.

► Account files are created and submitted electronically to a precollect letter service which sends out the letters and then sends a file back to post activity.

► Accounts ready to be sent to a collection agency are created and submitted to an agency. Payments and other transactions are then sent back and posted electronically to your system.

Now wouldn't that be great. Think of all the hours and days your staff spends on these activities. If you were able to reclaim those hours, what activities would you have them do — more insurance and self-pay follow-up? Spending more time on patient education? Or maybe just being able to keep up with current workloads in all areas?

Every one of these "possibilities" is available to 'Our Practice' today. It is not a futuristic vision. The practice that takes advantage of the electronic world is rewarded by expedited cash flows, lower costs through productivity, enhanced accuracy of data and top-of-the-line patient service.

This key step will examine the electronic world and help you maximize your current system. First, let us examine the different technologies which 'Our Practice' might consider.

Electronic eligibility systems

The technology exists to automatically create a file of the subscriber's insurance information, which is transmitted via modem to the insurance company's database. Eligibility and benefit level information is then transmitted back to the practice, identifying any problems.

Vendors exist which sell this technology. The problem is whether the insurance companies are allowing access to their databases. Each payer is at different stages in their evolution, some are "state-of-the-art," some allow "look-ups" on individual accounts, some use phone menu systems and others — those still in the dark ages — insist on "the next available representative" phone call.

Contact your major payers and ask them at what stage they are. If they have a system, which advances what you are doing now — take advantage of it. Ask them to describe what you or your system vendor need to do to implement. Also contact a vendor selling eligibility verification systems and hear what they offer and at what cost. It can't hurt to listen. It is in your and their best interests — for cost, productivity and provider satisfaction — to use this technology.

Electronic claims submission (ECS)

If you do nothing else in the world of Electronic Data Interchange (EDI), implement ECS with as many payers as you possibly can. The ability to download files and submit them to the payer — untouched by human hands — has been around for over a decade. Claim clearinghouses exist that accept claims for multiple insurance plans with distribution to the payers. Your practice management software vendor may have established partnerships with payers and clearinghouses which allow easy (and quick) implementation.

ECS has been the greatest boost to productivity in the last twenty years. Most practices use ECS for at least some payers — most notably Medicare. It should be used for as many payers as possible. Not only does it enhance productivity, it accelerates the turnaround of cash (over paper claims) by 15-45 days.

Using electronic claims also provides an invaluable control: the verification by the payer that the claims have been received. Unless they "blow-out" the file, the infamous "...there is no record of your claim having been received..." statement should not be uttered from the payer. Be sure to create back-ups of your sub- missions for at least 60 days. In the event they "blow-out" the file, you can resubmit the entire file. In addition, verify daily that the file has been received and is in process. In the instance of the clearinghouse, you will need to verify that the clearinghouse has received the file, and also that the *payer* has received the file — a verification process the clearinghouse should offer.

Electronic remittance advice (ERA)

Electronic remittance advice technology is the second greatest boost to productivity a practice can implement. Insurance companies have been slower to accommodate ERA for physician practices than hospitals but they are finally getting on board.

In this EDI activity, an electronic remittance is created by the payer and is transmitted to the provider. The provider captures this file, edits it against their patient account files and then posts it to the accounts. Exception reports are created which detail credit balances, unidentified accounts and payments which vary from expected payments.

The process should begin with a survey of all major payers to see if they create electronic files and the what format they will be submitting to the provider. The implementation of this system can be facilitated in many instances by the practice management software vendor. They will take a test file and "map" it out against their file specifications. Contact the vendor to investigate their capabilities.

The implementation process usually entails coordinating the payer's technology personnel with the vendor technology personnel. Once they start talking, to each other, the role of the practice will be to test the system prior to "going live."

Collection agency transaction interfaces

When investigating a collection agency "Our Practice" should make sure they are able to receive referred accounts electronically. Unless the agency is "old line" they will have this capability. The use of the electronic submission of accounts will free staff from processing reports and delays in account placements.

In this system, a file is created for accounts that have been reclassified to bad debt. This file will be transmitted to the agency. The agency will then map it out to their system. Additionally, all account transaction (payments and cancellations) will be transmitted as they occur. The agency, in turn, will transmit to "Our Practice's" system all account activity. "Our practice's" vendor information services staff will then map out the file to your system. The beauty of this approach is the immediate updating of account information. Payments received at the practice will alert the agency to cease further collection activity.

Survey your current agency(s) for its capabilities. Here is where "Our Practice" can lay the burden of implementation on the agency to facilitate this process and to work with the vendor or information services personnel.

Other electronic opportunities

Two other opportunities that you need to investigate are electronic interfaces to the precollection letter service and outsourcing your statement processing via electronic submission. The electronic interface to the precollection services will depend on the capabilities of the vendor. For outsourcing your statement processing, it will depend on a cost justification and how thin the internal resources are stretched.

Precollect letter service

The precollection letter service ideally has created working partnerships with "Our Practice's" software vendor to make this implementation feasible. If that is the case, "Our Practice's" system would be "profiled" in your statement processing cycle, with a file created for accounts which have received a certain number of statements. The internal statement processing would be suspended and a memo posted that the account has been referred to the precollect letter service. Both activities would be system generated. The file would be transferred electronically. Account transactions (cash payments and cancellations) would be transmitted. The precollect service would transmit activity and the information would be posted to "Our Practice's" system.

Outsourcing statement processing

This may be an opportunity if the printing, folding, stuffing, posting and mailing of statements are a burden on your staffs' time. If this activity keeps them from account management and other critical activities, this is definitely a function that needs to be outsourced.

Vendors dedicated to this activity are able to perform this activity at a relatively low cost. Print files are created which are submitted electronically to the vendor. Memos are posted and transaction information communicated between you and the vendor — much in the way of the precollect service.

Contact the vendors and cost justify based on the internal resources now used and how you would re-distribute the staffs' time resulting in enhanced cash flow and patient service. A word of caution — as with every vendor service — be sure the outsourced mail services are meeting your expectations of timely processing and delivery.

Get the most out of practice management software

Aside from the opportunities in the EDI world, make sure you are using the full power of your practice management software. What keeps many practices from using their system to its full potential is the initial profile and table setup. It will take someone who is:

➤ Motivated to learn the system's capabilities

➤ Detail orientated enough to become an expert at the profiles and tables

➤ Tenacious enough to implement

The payoff is worth it. It is a mission which, when accomplished, pays off in productivity, data accuracy and cash flow on a daily basis — week after week, month after month, year after year.

Prebill edits

Use the edits in your system to find out claims problems before they are submitted. Define the payer requirements and then try to have edits tight enough to mirror the payer's edits.

In addition, use the edit reports to define ongoing, persistent, internal data collection problems. Identify the errors that have the greatest impact on cash. Select the number one problem, identify the root causes and then formulate and implement a training session or system fix around the error. Once completed, take the second most damaging error and repeat the process. Do not try to fix everything all at once. Focus your energies on one problem at a time.

Contractual reimbursement master (CRM)

The use of the system's contractual reimbursement master is a system opportunity of which very few practices take advantage (assuming their management practice software has this capability). "Our Practice" is no exception. The CRM automatically "writes down" the receivable to the contractual amount at the time of billing. Most practices will wait for payment and the explanation of benefit (EOB) before writing off the contractual allowance.

Here is how the CRM operates. At the time of billing, the system will look for the CRM file (every software vendor uses a different name for this file — reimbursement master, contract master, managed care master,) which contains the contract terms. It will then use this file to:

➤ Estimate the payment

➤ Post the difference between the expected amount and charges to an allowance account

➤ Post the expected amount to the account

➤ Memo the account identifying the different activities

The ability to state the account and the overall receivables at "expected cash," enables the tight monitoring of all managed care contracts. It enables better receivable management through stating the accounts receivable at its true cash value.

The construction of a thorough CRM is time consuming, especially if the contract is fee based. In the case of fee-based contracts, do not attempt to input the entire CPT-4 list. Ask for a report identifying the top 200 charges of "Our Practice." In most cases (unless "Our Practice" is a multi-specialty clinic), the list will become insignificant after 50 service codes. These are the services that you will input into your CRM. All other services provided will be "residual" and not be monitored because of immateriality. (**Note of caution:** *if "Our Practice" provides a high cost service or supply — even if rarely — put this in the CRM just to be safe.*) For "discount off of charges," capitated or global fee reimbursement schemes, these will be more easily set up and maintained in your system.

Review each of your contract terms. Review with your vendor the process to implement and then test with one of "Our Practice's" lower impact payers. Once you feel comfortable with the results, move onto an implementation schedule with other major payers.

Employer master and insurance master

Different practice management systems may use different architecture, but there will be file tables that contain employer information and insurance plan information. When a patient is preregistered and describes their employer and insurance plan, the employer master, working in conjunction with the insurance master, will identify the exact plan and describe the benefit level. After verification with the patient, this information will save the registration staff "keystrokes" by automatically filling in the exact plan name, plan number and billing address.

By profiling employers' and the insurance plan benefits — information that is necessary to estimate the patient's liability, patient education on the expectation of payment at the time of service, and the exact amount — can be conducted.

To set up these files properly, "Our Practice" will need to contact the major employers in the area to find out which plans they are offering and the benefit levels of each of the plans. On a yearly basis (or whenever the employer changes insurance companies) "Our Practice" will need to make contact with the benefits manager of the company to update "Our Practice's" files.

The set up time for these tables is time consuming. The benefits of utilizing the employer and insurance masters are accuracy of data (cash flow), immediacy of data (for patient education) and patient service (being able to explain to them their insurance plan).

Collector's tools

If "Our Practice's" system has a collector's workstation, workfile or other paper collection tool, define it and then use it. It is the best organizing and prioritizing tool available for the collection staff.

The workstation is nothing more than a daily worklist created for a specific collector. Each day a list appears on the collector's screen for accounts that are in need of attention. The profiles can be set by payer, dollar amount, aging, alpha-split, etc. Additionally, management reports are created which supervisors will use to see the collector's efficiency (quantity) and effectiveness (quality).

The accounts in each of the collector's queue needs to monitored to ensure backlogs are not being created. Unless the collector takes an action on an account, the account will show up every day.

The creation of the profiles should not be a time consuming activity.

SUMMARY OF KEY ACTION STEP 10

► **Electronic technology is available which must be used to maximize cash flow, increase productivity and enhance patient education and service.**

- ❑ **Claims eligibility**
- ❑ **Claims submission**
- ❑ **Remittance posting**
- ❑ **Collection agency transactions**
- ❑ **Bill and statement processing**
- ❑ **Precollect letter transactions**

► **Electronic claims submission is the first system which needs to be implemented because it has an immediate impact on cash flow.**

► **The current practice management software functionality must be utilized:**

- ❑ **Prebill edits**
- ❑ **CRM**
- ❑ **Employer and insurance master**
- ❑ **Collector's tools**

To Do List

❑ Call system vendors and research system needs and their payer "relationships" for electronic claims submissions and remittance posting.

❑ Talk to payers and research their capabilities in accepting electronic claims submission and transmitting electronic remittance advices.

❑ Identify a major payer to implement for claims submission.

❑ Talk to your collection agency about exchanging electronic transaction data.

❑ Review the CRM capabilities of your system.

❑ Review the collection capabilities of your system.

Answer These Questions About "Our Practice":

❑ Are your staffs' workloads overwhelming? Where are the backlogs — billing? cash application? referring accounts to collection?

❑ Are you taking advantage of existing EDI technology? What are your peers in other practices doing to keep up with increasing volumes?

❑ Are you concerned that your managed care contract partners are paying according to contract terms? Do you manually audit their payments?   Do you use the CRM module?

Key Action Step 11
FORMAL TRAINING PROGRAM

A formal training program for new hires, as well as existing staff, is desired by all but accomplished by few. Unless you are a large practice with a training program staffed by professional trainers, it is probable there is no formal training at all. Most practices employ the "ask the person sitting next to you" approach to training.

The benefits of formal training are well documented: consistent application of policy and procedures, productivity, confidence in dealing with the public and employee confidence (with its corollaries of job satisfaction and employee retention).

"Our Practice" does not have the luxury of having staff dedicated to the training program. For this, the practice administrator (who has limited resources and time) must use her imagination in implementing (and probably doing the training) for new hires. The first action she takes is approaching the clinical leader of the practice to "co-champion" the training. With the clinical leader aware of the effort and the benefits enjoyed, the chance for successful implementation increase significantly.

This key action step is geared to designing and implementing a formal training program where time and expertise to develop lesson plans, instructional materials and trainers is limited.

Don't bite off more than you can chew

The first order of business is to decide on the set of "course offerings." Think in terms of the major categories of necessary education that will impact on cash flow, patient relations and cost. These endeavors can be described as getting bills and statements out accurately, meeting and exceeding workload standards and having your staff exhibit behaviors to the patients that will make their visits enjoyable.

Exhibit 11.1 Recommended base curriculum with the benefit area

Course	Benefit
1. The big picture and your role — A course on how a practice functions with special emphasis on the revenue cycle.	Cash Cost Patient relations
3. Putting the patient first	Patient relations
2. Practice management software training with functional training	Cash Productivity

Limit yourself to courses that your practice needs. There will be a tendency to try to develop an all encompassing program that attempts to tell everything about everything. *Resist the temptation.*

1. The big picture and your role in it

This course is a general overview of the practice with emphasis on the revenue cycle. The participant should be presented with a framework of the "what," the "why" and the "when" and their role within the system. In this way the employee is able to categorize all subsequent information in a logical structure.

Course content:

▶ **The revenue cycle from scheduling to zero balance.** Take each critical control point (scheduling, preregistration, insurance verification, reception/registration, time-of-service collections, billing, coding and account follow-up) and — from a high level perspective — explain the process.

▶ **The role of patient relations.** Explain the behaviors, which the practice requires of its employees and what to do with "difficult patients."

▶ **A glossary of terms.** Begin the process of acquainting the employee with the vocabulary of health care economics. Assume the participant knows nothing. When explaining a concept, be sure to explain terms.

▶ **Expectations for success.** Explain to the participants the goals and the goal setting process — both group and individual goals. Explain to them the feedback process which will keep them aware of their progress.

▶ **Policy and procedure review.** Make the participants aware they need to be knowledgeable with policies and procedures and their execution. Briefly review the most critical of these.

▶ **Receivable reports overview.** Review with participants the accounts receivable reports for account follow-up and accounts receivable management. Do not use this time to explain peripheral issues (such as how to fill out their timecard or vacation policy).

Classroom time involved: No more than four hours in two-hour segments.

▶ **When:** Given the second day, one session in morning, one session in afternoon.

- ➤ **Where:** Classroom, removed from distractions.
- ➤ **Prerequisite:** None.

2. Putting the patient first

Course is designed to give participant an understanding of public relations and the practice's philosophy. Participant will be schooled on the human relation's equation:

$$\text{Human Relations} = \text{Self} + \text{Other} + \text{Situation}$$

Sessions should be highly interactive with significant time spent on role playing.

Course content:

- ➤ Understanding of self through personality profiling
- ➤ Understanding of the other person
- ➤ Understanding the situations they will encounter
- ➤ Listening techniques and interviewing techniques
- ➤ How to deal with difficult people
- ➤ Practice's patient relations goals, scripts and role play. This will be on going training over the first month of employment.

Classroom time involved: This will be on going training over the first months of employment.

Eight hours spread out over a two-week period. The gaps will allow participants to test out techniques in live situations and bring back to the group their experiences. This session should be highly interactive.

- ➤ **When:** Initial session given on third day. Initial session should be a two-hour session on third day — two sessions: one in morning, one in afternoon. Subsequent sessions should be given in two-hour segments.
- ➤ **Where:** Classroom, removed from distractions.
- ➤ **Prerequisite:** Big picture

3. Practice management software training

Course is designed to give the participant a solid foundation in all aspects of the system. To facilitate understanding, cross training and promotions this is critical and will further emphasize how their role functions in coordination with the whole.

Course content:

- ➤ How to access computer with log-on procedures
- ➤ Menu review Review of each module
- ➤ Hands on practice with all on-line activities
  - ❑ Scheduling registration

- ❏ Insurance verification
- ❏ Collections-insurance and self-pay
▶ Coding System's report review

Classroom time involved: This will be on going training over the first month of employment. Initial session should be a four-hour session on third day — two sessions: one in morning, one in afternoon. Each hands-on session, depending on the topic, will be from 2-3 hours long. Each incremental session would be followed by a week of "live" training for at least a week per module.

- ▶ **When:** Initial session given on third day. Follow-up "hands-on" sessions should be followed up with "live" situation. Employee should be rotated through entire system for a week at time.
- ▶ **Where:** Classroom, removed from distractions.
- ▶ **Prerequisite:** Big picture and Putting the patient first

Developing course content and the lesson plan

The content exists, albeit in an unorganized fashion. It is up to you to identify, organize and document the necessary information. The way to begin is with the lesson plan.

The lesson plan is a sequential outline of the course which details what topics are being covered, what instructional aids are used, what reference handouts will be distributed, the medium used during each topic discussion (group discussion, lecture, exercise) and the length of each topic discussion. Use this document as a planning tool. Your first draft is a brainstorming session that will identify the topics that will be covered and a list of talking points. The topics will probably focus mainly on those activities you feel are in need of improvement.

Exhibit 11.2 is an example of a lesson plan. The final product of a lesson plan will be a document, which provides a detailed road map of who, what and when.

Exhibit 11.2 Example of a lesson plan

Course Title: The big picture
Session 1
Time: 2 hours
Location: Conference room
Equipment needed: ☐ Overhead ☐ PowerPoint Projector ☐ Flipchart ☐ Screen ☐ Other

Topic - Material	Time	Medium	Aides	Reference - Handouts
Introduction: "Welcome, in this session, we will be reviewing the critical functions of the revenue cycle with special emphasis..."	5 minutes	Overhead of agenda		Agenda
"First let's take a little test on our undertanding of the mission of the practice — at the end of the course, we will test ourselves again to see if..."	15 minutes	Test with group discussion		10 question quiz on students' understanding of group practice and the importance of accounts receivable cycle
"Lets go through the entire revenue cycle and examine why they are required and "Our Practice's" philosophy concerning...."	30 minutes	Overhead of revenue cycle	Revenue cycle chart for reference. Place on wall	
etc....				

The initial draft of your lesson plan will identify the topics to cover. This will lead your investigation into identifying the materials to further develop the topics. As these materials are accumulated, it will give form to the length of time necessary, the format, the instructional material and the reference aids.

Accumulating the material

Start collecting existing training materials. You will take the existing documentation and organize them under your main topic categories. These would include:

> **Policy and procedures.** Review these documents to see if they accurately reflect the current or evolving philosophy of the practice. The main document will be the credit and collection policy. Does it address such issues as expectation of time-of-service payment, alternative financing options and the write-off to bad debt parameters including the statement cycle process. Other policy and procedure documents would include:

> ❏ Scheduling procedures
> ❏ Registration procedures
> ❏ Insurance verification procedures
> ❏ The missing ticket (Charge) procedures
> ❏ Billing processes
> ❏ Collection procedures

> **Contract and payer-provided documentation.** Part of the reference material you will be handing out to staff are portions of payer contracts which address utilization guidelines, payment term, reimbursement terms and other pertinent sections which "Our Practice's" staff need to know to perform their jobs.

> **Interview of staff.** This is an excellent method to find out what is happening currently on the front lines. Sit down with each person (or the lead person) and document how they perform their tasks. This is not the time to do performance improvement initiatives. You need to listen and document, even though you might not like what you're hearing.

> Ask staff for the documentation they use; there probably will be a hodge-podge of "cheat-sheets," yellow sticky tabs and the like. Copy what documentation you can and document the rest. This is also a good time to start identifying "screens" in the automated system which you will want to print as an instructional tool.

> **Patient communications.** Collect patient brochures, copies of statements and any aids the self-pay collectors use when talking with the patients.

> **Vendor information.** Hopefully your practice management software vendor has provided a good "how-to" manual. If not, call them and ask if they have an instructional manual. They should have something which

staff can use to train. Review the manuals. Your task is to create brief step-by-step instructions — the less text the better.

Also contact other vendors with whom you do business and collect any materials which help you define their product and provide instructions on its use. Examples would be collection agency, precollect letter service, prebill edit product and alternative financing partners.

➤ **Books and articles.** Especially in planning for the courses with "The big picture and putting the patient first," there are books and publications (such as MGMA's *Putting the Patient First: Up-front with Advocacy and Community Service* by Bob Richards and Jeanan Yasiri) which will make development of these courses easier. They will aid not only in developing course content but you may also make a required reading list for all employees. For more information on MGMA publications, visit the online catalog at **http://www.mgma.com.**

As you go through the documentation, it will prompt further development of your lesson plan. The next step is organize the information and develop a presentation-quality training session.

Information overload-creating the presentation

You now should have too much information. Step back from the process and see the training from the point of view a new hire. In the initial stage they will be able to handle only the big picture or the very little picture ("here, do this and only this, over and over"). The shape of the course should be enough information to make the student increasingly confident in their skills and more productive in the shortest amount of time. Too much information and they will be overwhelmed and stop learning.

Categorize the information into their respective course and then into their functional areas. Review the material and then compare it to your lesson plan. Does the information fit within the scope of the lesson plan? Should it? Is the student ready for this material or does it come under the "overwhelmed" category? Be ruthless. In training, less is usually more. Avoid exceptions to the rule like the plague. The student is not ready for exceptions and will feel overwhelmed. When this happens the learning process stops.

Build the course through the lesson plan. Outline the talking points, annotate where instructional material will be used and, if you are going to use overhead screens, identify which screen. If you feel it is necessary, script out the dialogue.

The lesson plan is a work in progress. As it "comes to life," you will modify it, find gaps, need more research and discover inventive ways to present it.

As you build the lesson plan think about these...

- ▶ **Quizzes.** It is a good idea to quiz the student. These quizzes should be short, hit the highlights and be used to review each segment of the course.

- ▶ **Videos.** There are a host of videos out there on customer service. This is an inexpensive, entertaining way to get a point across. It also breaks up the day. Use as a vehicle to encourage group discussions on how you can implement at "Our Practice."

- ▶ **Flip charts.** Use flip charts during group discussions to document the groups' thought. This will underline how you value their input. Do not make value judgements on the worth of their comments. Document all the points.

- ▶ **Final examination with certification.** There is something to be said for having worked and struggled, achieved and then be recognized for your performance. Give a final exam for all key areas in which the person will be involved — let them take it as many times as necessary — then award them a certificate of achievement. The certificate would bear the name of the practice, the proficiency demonstrated and signed by a physician, the instructor and anyone else which would demonstrate the practice appreciates the students effort.

Lights, camera, action! — The presentation

The hard fact of presentations is the more you do the better you get. Expect the first few outings to be "learning experiences." The first few presentations will highlight material which is too in depth, inappropriate for new staff, unclear or in need of better examples.

- ▶ **No distractions.** Make sure the setting for training is conducive to learning — no distractions. Make sure your staff knows there is no reason for interruptions unless it's a true emergency.

- ▶ **Confidence.** If you are uncomfortable with formal presentations, read a book on effective presentations and gaining confidence. But confidence comes from doing — and sometimes doing poorly. Just keep after it, you will get better.

- ▶ **Keep making it better.** Once you have the base product, it becomes easier to improve! Maybe you will want to add a whole new module to an already existing course. Keep the course work dynamic — changing as your practice changes.

- ▶ **Get others involved in teaching.** Nothing makes you learn faster and better than having to teach a subject. You have staff that will be motivated to teach. Let them demonstrate their expertise by teaching others.

- ▶ **Use the certification program to promote and reward.** The student who demonstrates proficiency by "graduating" from each course adds value to the practice. Consider the idea of promoting the achiever through a structured title and wage enhancement. The wage increase does not have to be large to be effective. Enhanced job titles are without cost. Use them to show appreciation.

▶ **Outside training.** There are outside seminars that your staff needs to attend. If a professional organization is giving a course on Medicare billing, a member of your staff should attend. Make it the responsibility of the attendee to present to the rest of the group a mini training session on the subject. By sending different staff to programs, it allows the student to see the bigger picture by coming in contact with their peer group. It also shows your trust, appreciation and willingness to invest in their professional development.

▶ **Yearly refresher classes.** Make sure to have yearly "refresher" classes for all. This will keep everyone current, including yourself.

▶ **Have Fun.** This should be informative and fun for both the student and you.

SUMMARY OF KEY ACTION STEP 11

▶ **Training is crucial to success by impacting cash, productivity and patient satisfaction.**

▶ **Enlist the aid of the clinical leader of your practice to co-champion the project.**

▶ **Limit your training to the critical impact points.**

  ❑ **The big picture**
  ❑ **System software training**
  ❑ **Patient relations expectations**

▶ **Create a formal presentation with on-the-job reference material.**

▶ **Enlist your vendors in providing training.**

▶ **Use outside materials to aid in the presentation.**

▶ **Complement staff training by staffing individual staff members to seminars on specific topics.**

To Do List

- ❑ Approach the clinical leader of your practice and tell her of the need and your ideas for a formal training program.

- ❑ Identify the area most in need of a formal training session.

- ❑ Call system vendor for documentation in system training.

- ❑ Collect policy and procedures. Interview staff.

Answer These Questions About "Our Practice":

- ❑ When someone is hired, how much time is expended on their training before they come in contact with patients?

- ❑ Do each of your staff members understand the importance of all the activities in the revenue cycle?

- ❑ Do they understand why their role is so important?

- ❑ Are you frustrated with your staffs' seeming inability to make sound decisions? If so, why do you think this is?

Key Action Step 12
THE IMPLEMENTATION PLAN AND MOTIVATION FOR RESULTS

Everything "Our Practice" has done up to this point will come to nothing if it does not execute its strategies and involves staff in the process. If one day out of the blue you announce all the wonderful things you have in store for them without preparing a motivational environment for staff, the system and you will fail. This final chapter lays out a sequence of events that must occur to implement changes and how to create the climate for motivation and success.

Communicate! Communicate! Communicate!

The first order of business is to communicate how the system needs to change, why it's important to the financial viability of the practice and each staff member's role. This process should be taken seriously. Each area of change needs to be detailed, the benefits listed, the action plan explained and how each individual will be involved. Do a formal presentation. Nothing less will do.

The financials

Begin with the financial picture of the current receivables. (See Key Action Step 1.)

- ► **The "Cash Gap."** Trend the net revenue and cash collected over the last six months. Explain the need for the two trend lines to be identical. Show that for the receivables to be set right, the "cash collected" line needs to exceed the "net revenue" line for the next six months.

- ► **DRO.** Layout the Day's Revenue Outstanding and compare them to the best performing practices and to the average performing practices. Explain the amount of dollars bound up in the receivable between "Our Practice" and the best and average practices.

- ► **Bad debt.** Again compare "Our Practice" to the best and the average. Show the dollar impact on the bottom line for each 1/4 percent decrease in the bad debt to revenue.

- ► **Dollars over 90 days percent.** Do the comparisons and explain this is an indication of the failure of the system. Trace this back to the DRO and the dollars involved.

Display the cash, DRO, bad debt and dollars over 90 days and percent goals for the next six months. Emphasize the goals are attainable and are being achieved by the top performing practices. Let this statement lead into a discussion of how these practices are attaining success — the best practices model.

The best practices model

It is at this point that you will need to take the team through a discussion on the receivables demonstrated by the best performing practices. Describe the revenue and describe what key functions need to occur, why they need to occur and the impact each has on cash and customer service. The best practice model you will use is the information provided in Key Action Steps 2-9.

During this process allow time for concerns from staff about the changes which are necessary to execute the action plan. Look for ideas from staff about how to improve the implementation of the plan within the overriding structure. However, keep reiterating the importance of the key control and why it is necessary to implement the entire strategy.

The action plan

The action plan lists events that must occur, states when they must occur and who is responsible for the events. Make sure that the plan is sufficiently detailed to include all necessary steps in the process. The action plan is a dynamic document which will change as obstacles are encountered or an omitted step is discovered. (See figure 12.1.)

Exhibit 12.1 Excerpt from an action plan

Step	Activity	Start	End	Action Person
1	**COMMUNICATE TIME OF SERVICE (TOS) PAYMENT EXPECTATION**			
1.1	**Review credit & collection policy**	1/1/99	1/5/99	Jodi
1.2	**Draft "request for payment" scripts for preregistration personnel**			
1.21	☐ Identify possible patient "objection" to TOS payment	1/1		Susan
1.22	☐ Draft scripts for "objections"	1/1		Susan
1.3	**Prepare listing of payment alternative**			
1.31	☐ Document under what circumstances alternative would be available	1/1		Bobbi
1.32	☐ Prepare scripts for preregistration personnel on alternative financing options			Bobbi
1.4	**Training**			
1.41	☐ Prepare training documentation	1/15	1/30	Susan
1.42	☐ Prepare certification test	1/15	1/30	Bobbi
1.43	☐ Schedule training			Bobbi/Susan
1.43	☐ Conduct training			Bobbi/Susan
1.44	☐ Administer certification test			Bobbi/Susan
1.45	☐ Award certifications			Bobbi/Susan

Take the time with your staff to go over the action plan line item by line item. Encourage feedback to discover sequencing problems, too aggressive (or too soft) timeframes, missing steps or obstacles that need to be addressed and built into the action plan.

The action plan is the document that will remind everyone of the critical actions that must be taken. During the implementation stage, when confusion reigns, regroup the team, review the action plan, change as dictated by the situation and then keep moving forward.

Make sure the action plan does not overwhelm staff. Make sure the sequencing of events occurs in an orderly fashion with the largest payback items happening prior to smaller ones. To ensure quality data collection, customer service and cash collections most likely your energies will focus on front-end processes. It is also probable, if your receivables are out of control, you will develop an immediate strategy(s) for a cash acceleration clean-up project.

Exhibit 12.2 Success factors for the action plan

❑ Make sure the action plan does not overwhelm staff.

❑ Make sure the sequencing of events occurs in an orderly fashion.

❑ Orchestrate the plan to have largest payback items occurring first. A major victory early will drive future successes.

❑ Take the time to detail all the main action steps. A well documented plan will save time and frustration during implementation.

❑ Get as many — if not all — of your staffs' names on the action plan.

❑ Make the schedule tight but allow a little more time up front to allow staff to get comfortable with the process. A project, which begins with everyone missing the first deadline, is a dead project.

❑ Allow for slippage in the schedule. Be prepared for the unexpected or unforeseen obstacles to change the timelines.

Goal setting

Individual goal setting is critical in the overall success of the project and to the success of the individual. It is also one of the four main ingredients in the motivational environment:

➤ Staff involved in decision making which impacts their role

➤ Staff having access to information which impacts their role

► Staff aware of practice's goal and their individual goals

► Celebrating successes

Without goals, a staff member is forever unsure of whether they are successful or not. This reduces job satisfaction and increases stress. An individual with goals will be able to work towards that goal and, when accomplished, will take pride in the accomplishment and feel secure in their competency.

Goal setting will occur after the rollout of the overall goals and action plan. The process steps are:

► Identify key performance areas.

► Develop key performance indicators for each key performance area.

► Set short-range goals.

► Develop a strategic action plan for short-range goals.

► Set long range goals.

► Develop a strategic action plan for long range goals.

The process is a simple, effective map for individual and team goal setting, and is highly effective in cash management.

Identify key performance areas. To prompt your thinking, review job descriptions. Identify and note the areas of responsibility in each job description. Add to this list key performance areas which are missing from the job descriptions, but you have identified as critical. If no written job description exists, responsibilities as they are understood should be described in writing.

List the responsibilities under each key performance area. Use one to four words to describe each area. Examples: cash flow, staff development, bad debt, budget, collections, self-development, quality control, agency placements, billings, expenses, patient relations, registrations, job enrichment. The key performance areas should be:

► Directly associated with overall objectives

► Within the authorities of a specific position

Collectively, the list must include the major control points of the revenue cycle.

Establish performance indicators. Identify a quantifiable performance standard for each performance indicator. Be specific. Ask yourself, "What indicator will provide an effective, quantifiable test of success?"

Some examples of individual/team performance indicators are:

► Percent of preregistered patients to total

► Percent of insurance verifications to total

- Percent of time-of-service collections to total "opportunities"
- Percent of charges over standard delay from service to charge input (2 days? 3 days?)
- Percent of prebill edit rejections
- Percent of payer bill edit rejections
- Average days from charge posting date to billing
- Number of resolved accounts per day per insurance collector
- Number of resolved accounts per day per self-pay collector

Exhibit 12.3   Set goals

Goals must be smart:
- **S**pecific
- **M**easurable
- **A**chievable
- **R**elevant

Before, during and after implementation

Maintain a visible presence for goals. Don't tuck the practice's revenue cycle goals away in a drawer. Post them (out of sight of patients but in a prominent place) so that everyone is reminded of why they are important to the process. Every month make a poster of your Cash goal target and track daily cash collections (an easily accomplished graphic is a thermometer, but use your imagination). Also track your monthly progress on *Day's Revenue Outstanding, Bad Debt Expense* and *Percent of Dollars Over 90 Days*.

Keep your staff informed. Over and above the practice's financial targets, keep your staff informed on all the individual/team goals. Group meetings are an excellent setting to review performance improvement and prompt discussions on obstacles to overcome and staff ideas for improvement.

Celebrate your successes. In the beginning, you may feel there is little to celebrate. But it's your job to find the successes. Did time-of-service collections improve by even one percent this month? Celebrate. Did your collection follow-up team make more contacts this week than the prior week? Celebrate. Find something positive about each of your teams and CELEBRATE. Punctuate the celebration with small gifts (movie tickets and other small, fun gifts).

One reason for a major celebration is when the major financial indicators of the practice have been accomplished for the month. It is then time to bring everyone together to emphasize the importance of the goal. The physicians (or a physician representative) should be in attendance and a personal message of appreciation delivered. This would be a good time for a social time with food and a chance to bask in the warm glow of success.

Celebrations need not be big nor the small gifts expensive. The true motivational gift comes when a team comes together to appreciate each other and to have the team appreciated by an objective, respected source (i.e., the physician).

When successes have been accomplished and the team understands the goals are within reach, and that the reaching of these goals is important and appreciated, success becomes addictive.

SUMMARY OF KEY ACTION STEP 12

▶ **Communicate your practice's financial goals.**

▶ **Communicate individual goals.**

▶ **Communicate the Action Plan.**

▶ **Communicate progress towards the goals.**

▶ **Celebrate successes.**

▶ **Involve everyone in the decision-making process.**

▶ **Include everyone in the information loop.**

To Do List

- ❑ **Establish practice goals**

- ❑ **Establish individual goals by function**

- ❑ **Design posters for displaying progress towards goals**

- ❑ **Plan for celebrations of success**

Answer These Questions About "Our Practice":

- ❑ **When was the last time you celebrated a quantified success?**

- ❑ **Does each member of your staff have a goal and do they know how to attain it?**

- ❑ **Do you know when your efforts result in a success?**

- ❑ **Can you do what 'Our Practice' has done? (The answer is "Yes")**

- ❑ **Good luck!**

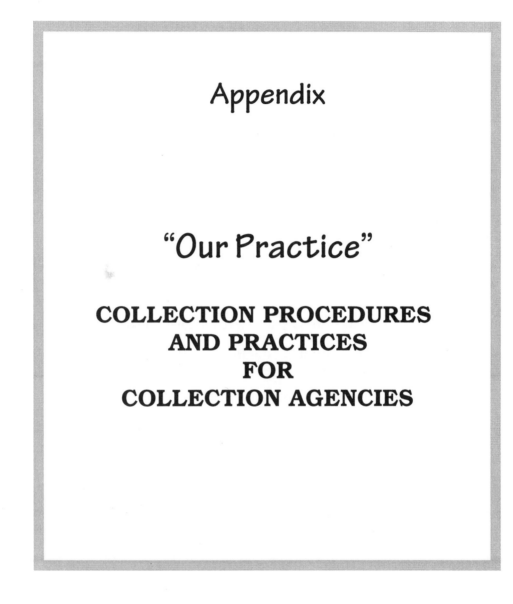

Appendix

"Our Practice"

COLLECTION PROCEDURES
AND PRACTICES
FOR
COLLECTION AGENCIES

Collection Procedures And Practices For Collection Agencies

The following Collection Procedures and Work Standards enable "Our Practice" to monitor, direct and measure the collection activity, recovery processes and performance of contracted collection agencies.

Basic requirements of the collection agency

1. Excellent reputation in the community (or communities) in which they operate with merchants, members of the medical profession and other clients

2. Compliance with state's regulatory requirements in bonds and licenses

3. Clean bill of health from Better Business Bureau and other consumer protection entities

4. In full compliance with policy and procedures of "Our Practice"

5. Will participate in "Our Practice's" goal setting process

6. Will help administer "Our Practice's" efforts in Financial Assistance Program

7. Will present collection effectiveness reports to "Our Practice's" management and staff

8. Will achieve most effective collection rate based on accounts placed

9. Will have made significant investment in technology

10. Management reports are flexible meeting information needs of "Our Practice"

Goal setting

A critical part of "Our Practice's" collection effectiveness program is goal setting. It is expected of the agency to be able to predict collection rates factoring in the following variables:

➤ Age of the account
➤ Dollar amount of balance

► Employment demographics

► Economics of service area

"Our Practice" should compare the collection effectiveness will be compared and of the agenicies it is currentlyusing. The result of this comparison should then be used for baseline setting and then goal setting. The comparison statistics will be based on the History and Analysis Management Report (see attachment). It is critical this report isolates actual cash collections from noncash categories (i.e., "close and return," bankruptcy, deceased, etc.).

The comparison reports will be shared with all agencies "Our Practice" continues to use. Because all agencies receive a like-type account distribution (alpha-split), an agency which does not compare favorably to its peer group will be given a period of time in which to improve. At the end of the period, if improvement is not demonstrated, the agency may be terminated.

Agencies will be asked to make quarterly presentations to staff collectors and supervisory personnel on their collection effectiveness and achievement of their goals.

Collection agency procedures

A. Data transmission

The collection agency of choice will be able to receive and transmit all transaction data via electronic transmission. All expenses associated with the set-up, implementation and maintenance would be the responsibility of the collection agency. Any expenses needed to modify, enhance or to integrate systems or networks are the responsibility of the agency.

Transmission of data will include the following:

► Transmission of account data for the purpose of account placement

► Transmission of account status, inventory and activity reports

► Transmission of remittance statements, inventory accounting, close and return reports, bankruptcy and legal account status

B. Systems utilization

The agency will maintain, upgrade and provide, at their expense, an adequate accounts receivable collection follow-up system. This system will include a predictive and/or auto-dialing system. The accounts receivable management system will provide:

► On line access to account status information

► Collector queue management

   ❑ Ability to assign dedicated collector queues

- ❏ Ability to list accounts by individual collector by account balance criteria and alpha split
- ► Account placement/volume control
  - ❏ Ability to handle large placement volumes
  - ❏ Systems account storage capability
- ► On site systems service representatives and programmers

C. Reporting and information services

The collection agency will provide the following reporting and information services:

- ► History & Analysis Report
- ► Account Activity Reports
  - ❏ Monthly Collector Activity Report
  - ❏ Monthly Call Activity Report
  - ❏ Monthly Close and Return Report
- ► Monthly Account Maintenance and Status Reports
  - ❏ Monthly Account Inventory Report
  - ❏ Monthly Account Status Report
  - ❏ Monthly Collection Performance Report
  - ❏ Monthly Deceased Close and Return report
  - ❏ Monthly Predictive Dialing/Auto-Dial Campaign Activity Report
  - ❏ Monthly Account Legal Status Report
  - ❏ Monthly Bankruptcy Report
  - ❏ Monthly Account Suspend Report
  - ❏ Monthly Claims Acknowledgement Report

D. Fee structures

The collection agency of choice will provide an equitable fee structure. It is recommended to entertain proposals based on:

- ► Age of account
- ► Precollect or other "value added" services
- ► Incentive fee structure based on collection effectiveness and complaints concerning agency

E. Staffing

The agency of choice will maintain an adequate number of well-trained collectors dedicated to the "Our Practice" accounts.

The agency will ensure all collectors are familiar with (and have been successfully tested on) the Fair Debt Collection Practices Act and the provisions of Title VIII.

F. Collection/recovery methods and techniques

The agency will incorporate the following collection methods:

1. Collector queue sizes

    ► Collector queues shall be no larger than 600 accounts per collector

2. Collection strategy

    ► All payments and correspondence must be directed to the collection agency of choice.

    ► All accounts must be paid in full within six months from date of placement or closed and returned unless approved by "Our Practice."

    ► No account will be referred for litigation by the agency of choice without prior suit authorization. The agency will pay for all legal, court and attorney fees. Agency will attempt to recoup collection expense of "Our Practice."

    ► All communications will be in compliance to local, state and federal regulations with regards to the Fair Debt Collection Practices laws and regulations.

    ► The agency will close and return, upon demand, any and all accounts recalled within forty-eight (48) hours of the return request.

    ► The agency account representatives will request payment in full unless one of the following situations arise:

        ❑ The guarantor disputes the account or a portion thereof. The guarantor is to pay any undisputed portion immediately and send the dispute in writing to "Our Practice."

        ❑ The guarantor proves to be unable to pay the balance in full. "Our Practice" will pre-authorize payment arrangements based on the Budget Plan Schedule (see Exhibit 1). All other payment arrangements must have specific approval from "Our Practice." Documentation substantiating the inability of the guarantor to pay will be available for audit purposes.

Exhibit 1 Budget plan schedule

Balance outstanding	Minimum payment	Preferred payment
$101 to $200	$ 50	Total
$201 to $300	$ 75	Total
$301 to $400	$ 75	$125
$401 to $500	$ 75	$125
$501 to $600	$100	$150
$601 to $700	$125	$175
$701 to $800	$125	$175
$901 to 1000	$150	$200
Over $1000	$175	$220
	"Our Practice" must approve if longer than six months	"Our Practice" must approve if longer than six months

3. Collection notices and letter series

   ➤ All collection notices and letter series will be approved by "Our Practice" prior to any communications.

   ➤ Local, state and federal regulatory agencies will have approved all communications.

4. Phone attempts

   ➤ All accounts listed (with the exception of "statement-only accounts [based on dollar amount]) will receive a telephone attempt within two (2) days of placement.

5. Legal activity

   ➤ No accounts listed shall be placed in a prelegal or legal status by the agency of choice without first meeting the following criteria:

      ❑ All standard collection attempts must be exhausted.

      ❑ Suit authorization must be obtained from "Our Practice."

      ❑ All attorneys utilized by the agency must be approved by "Our Practice."

      ❑ The agency shall, at their expense, pay all attorney, court costs and related expenses.

6. Patient relations

   ➤ The agency will abide by all local, state and federal collection regulations and statutes, and maintain the highest degree of decorum and debtor dignity and emphasize to its employees the need for consistent and productive patient relations.

G. Performance audits

▶ The agency will submit to open, on site performance audits without prior notice, either written or verbal.

H. Contract compliance

▶ The agency will abide by all stipulations delineated in contract by "Our Practice." Failure to comply with all contract stipulations will result in immediate termination.

I. Contract termination

▶ This is not an exclusive arrangement. "Our Practice" reserves the right to terminate any contractual agreements with the agency immediately by denying access to further accounts. All accounts at the agency will be returned to "Our Practice" within 60 days from the date of notification of termination.

J. Collection supervisor profile

▶ The collection supervisor should fit the following profile:

❑ As an agent of the medical group pracitce, they must conduct themselves in the best interests of "Our Practice."

❑ Have three to five years experience in the collections industry with emphasis in health care.

❑ Demonstrate ability to design programs which meet the customers needs.

❑ Be well versed in the collection technique and methodology of health care.

❑ Be aware of the patient relations mission of "Our Practice."

❑ Have to communicate collection agency processes to "Our Practice" managers and staff.

❑ Have above-average management skills.

K. Collector profile

In an effort to maintain the level of performance and productivity in reaching predetermined cash goals, the agency's collection personnel should fit the following profile:

▶ As an agent of the medical group practice, they must conduct themselves in the best interests of "Our Practice."

▶ Able to effectively persuade guarantor to pay bill within the guidelines of "Our Practice."

▶ Possess excellent listening skills.

▶ Has the ability to think clearly and quickly.

▶ Is resourceful, creative and dedicated.

- ▶ Possess excellent verbal communication skills.
- ▶ Ability to adapt quickly to various debtor personalities.
- ▶ Is professional in appearance and attitude.

INDEX

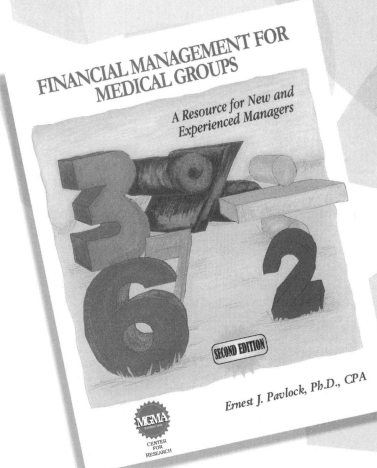
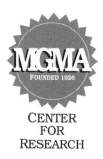

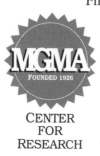

To order **MGMA publications** or to find out more about MGMA membership, just call toll-free **1-888-ASK-MGMA, ext. 888** **Monday - Friday 8:00 a.m. - 5:00 p.m. MST.** Or look for MGMA on-line at **http://www.mgma.com**